THE ULTIMATE GUIDE TO LASTING WEIGHT LOSS

Hilda Obi, DNP and Victor Obi, RPh
The Ultimate Guide to Lasting Weight Loss

Isbn: 979-8-89383-986-9

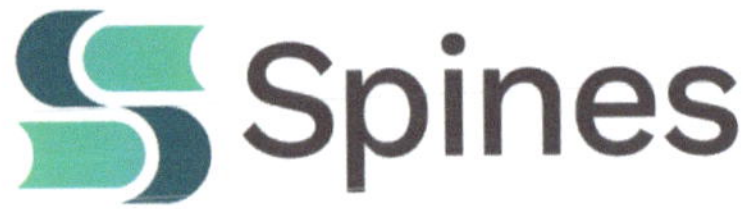

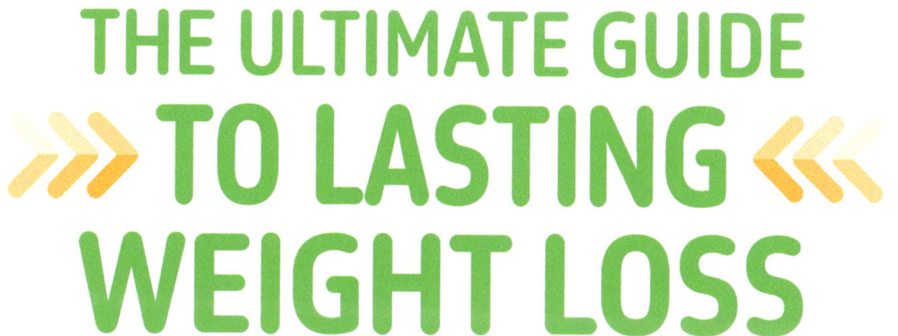

THE ULTIMATE GUIDE TO LASTING WEIGHT LOSS

Dr Hilda Obi

Acknowledgements

First and foremost, I want to express my deepest gratitude to my beloved husband, Victor Obi. Victor, your invaluable experience as a pharmacist in the pharmaceutical health and wellness industry has been instrumental in the creation of this book. Your insights, dedication, and unwavering support has made you an indispensable Co-author. Thank you for standing by my side and for your continuous encouragement.

A heartfelt thank you goes out to all my wonderful staff. Your unwavering support, hard work, and commitment to using this guide to educate the thousands of patients we've seen over the years are deeply appreciated. You are the backbone of our success, and your dedication makes a significant difference in the lives of those we serve.

To our amazing sons, Victor Jr and Michael, thank you for your continued support in all that we do. Your belief in our mission and your encouragement are sources of strength and inspiration. You motivate us to strive for excellence and to make a positive impact in the world.

Lastly, I extend my deepest appreciation to the incredible individuals who have trusted us and implemented this guide for their success all these years. Your dedication to your health and your belief in our methods are the driving forces behind our work. Thank you for allowing us to be a part of your journey towards a healthier and happier life.

With immense gratitude,

Dr. Hilda, DNP

Table of Contents

Introduction 9

Overview of the Ultimate Guide 11

How the Program works 13

Detox Phase 17

Smart Eating throughout the Program 19

Modified Ketogenic Phase 21

Regular Phase 21

Other Dietary Recommendations 23

Why you need to Stay well Hydrated 26

Importance of limiting Sugar and Salt 29

How to read a Food Label 32

Averting High Cholesterol 35

Incorporating Physical Activities 36

Behavior Modification for Weight Management 45

The Effects of Stress on the body 50

What has Sleep got to do with weight loss 53

Importance of Supplementation 56

Semaglutide and Tirzepatide: The Game Changers 60

Common side effects and how to manage them 66

The Power of GLP-1 and the Ultimate Guide 70

Why do you Plateau? 73

Other factors that affect your weight loss goals 79

Maintenance Phase to lasting Weight loss 82

Dining Out and On-the-Go Practical Tips 84

Healthy Fast-Foods and Snack Options 88

Conclusion: Your Path to lifelong Health and Wellness 91

Appendix A: Quick Start Guide 93

Appendix B: Two Week Low Carb Sample Menu 94

Appendix C: Two Week Spanish Sample Menu 98

Appendix D: Two Week Vegetarian Sample Menu 102

Appendix E: Healthy Salad Dressing Options 107

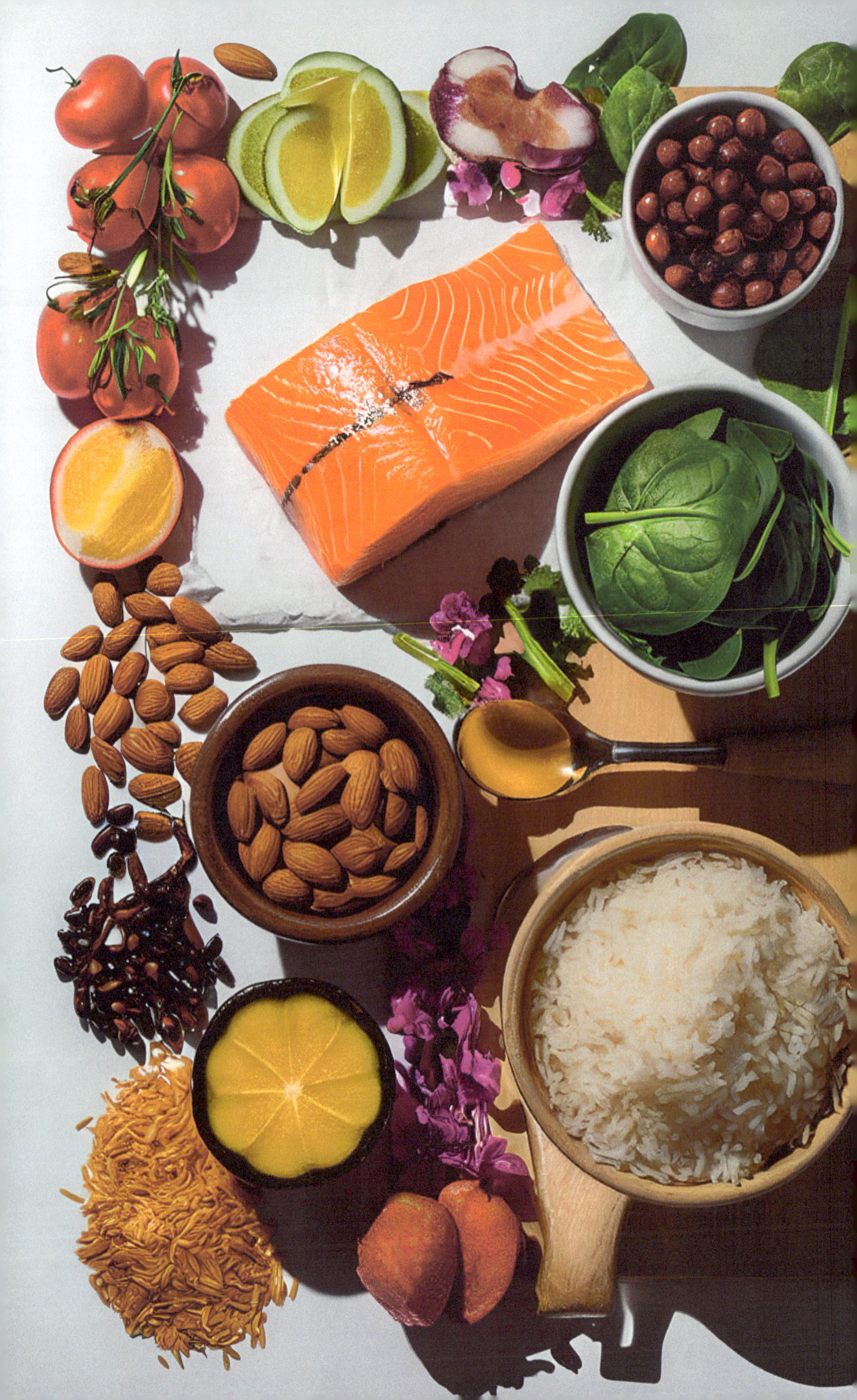

Embrace the Journey to a Healthier You

Welcome to "The Ultimate Guide to Lasting Weight Loss," where your journey to a healthier, happier, and more vibrant life begins. Imagine waking up each day with boundless energy, a renewed sense of confidence, and a body that feels strong and capable. This isn't just a dream—it's within your reach, and this guide is here to help you every step of the way.

In a world filled with fad diets, quick fixes, and endless promises, it's easy to feel overwhelmed and disheartened. But real, lasting weight loss isn't about deprivation or unrealistic goals. It's about making informed, sustainable changes that transform your life from the inside out. This guide is your comprehensive roadmap, based on my years of experience in my weight loss and wellness center as a certified expert in Obesity Medicine and a seasoned Doctor of Nursing Practice. I also serve as a Lifestyle and Wellness consultant. With my extensive experience, I have successfully helped thousands of patients achieve their weight loss goals and maintain their results.

Our program is divided into four distinct phases: Detox, Modified Ketogenic, Regular, and Maintenance. Each phase is carefully crafted to support your body's natural rhythms and needs, ensuring a smooth and effective journey toward your goals. From cleansing your body of toxins in the Detox Phase to building lifelong habits in the Maintenance Phase, you will find clear, actionable steps that guide you every step of the way.

But this guide is more than just a diet plan. It's a holistic approach that integrates the power of GLP-1, Glucagon Like Peptide-1 or Glucose-dependent Insulinotropic Polypeptide (GIP) Receptors a hormone that plays a crucial role in regulating appetite and metabolism. With the support of GLP-1, you can overcome plateaus and accelerate your progress, all under the guidance of experienced healthcare professionals.

We understand that life doesn't stop for weight loss. That's why we've included practical tips for dining out, managing occasional indulgences, and staying motivated when the going gets tough. You'll find strategies for overcoming plateaus, ensuring you remain on track even when faced with challenges. And to make your journey even more enjoyable, we've included sample menus that are both delicious and satisfying.

This is not just another diet book. It's a commitment to yourself, to your health, and to a future filled with possibilities. It's about embracing a new lifestyle, one that empowers you to live your best life. Every small change, every healthy choice, and every step forward brings you closer to the vibrant, energetic life you deserve.

So, are you ready to take the first step? To embrace the journey and transform your life? "The Ultimate Guide to Lasting Weight Loss" is here to guide, support, and inspire you. Together, we can achieve the extraordinary. Welcome to the beginning of your new life. Let's make it happen!

Overview of the Ultimate Guide

Welcome to "The Ultimate Guide to lasting Weight loss," Dr. Hilda's comprehensive weight loss guide designed to help you achieve your healthiest self through a balanced approach of diet, exercise, and behavior modification. This book is your key to unlocking the secrets of lasting weight loss, ensuring you not only shed those extra pounds but also embrace a healthier, happier lifestyle.

The Power of a Balanced Diet

Emphasis is placed on the importance of a balanced diet. This guide will show you how to make nutritious food choices that fuel your body while keeping you satisfied. By following the recommended meal plans and understanding the principles of healthy eating, you'll learn how to enjoy delicious, wholesome foods that promote weight loss and overall well-being. Imagine savoring vibrant salads, hearty whole grains, lean proteins, and fresh fruits, all while watching the numbers on the scale steadily decline. Additionally, you will learn healthy food options to select when dining out and foods to avoid.

The Importance of Regular Exercise

Dieting alone isn't enough to achieve your weight loss goals, which is why this "Ultimate Guide to lasting Weight loss" includes a comprehensive exercise program. Recommended exercise routines are designed to be effective, enjoyable, and adaptable to all fitness levels. Whether you're a beginner or a seasoned athlete, you'll find workouts that boost your metabolism, tone your muscles, and improve your cardiovascular health. Picture yourself feeling stronger, more energetic, and more confident as you progress and build endurance and intensity through these recommended exercises.

Incorporating the Power of GLP-1 (Semaglutide and Tirzepatide)

To accelerate your weight loss journey, Dr. Hilda introduces the power of GLP-1 (glucagon-like peptide-1) in "The Ultimate Guide to lasting Weight loss." GLP-1 is a naturally occurring hormone that plays a crucial role in appetite regulation and glucose metabolism. When harnessed correctly, GLP-1 can be a game-changer in achieving your weight loss goals sooner than you ever thought possible. Under Dr. Hilda's expert guidance, you'll learn how to incorporate GLP-1 into your regimen safely and effectively.

GLP-1 works by increasing feelings of fullness and reducing hunger, making it easier to adhere to a calorie-controlled diet. With the support of GLP-1, you'll find it less challenging to resist unhealthy cravings and portion sizes. This hormone also slows down gastric emptying, meaning you'll feel full for longer periods, further aiding in weight management. Additionally, GLP-1 helps regulate blood sugar levels, reducing the risk of type 2 diabetes—a common concern for those struggling with weight.

In "The Ultimate Guide to lasting Weight loss," Dr. Hilda provides detailed information on how GLP-1 can be utilized as part of a comprehensive weight loss strategy. She discusses the benefits of GLP-1 medications, which have been proven to support significant weight loss when combined with a healthy diet and regular exercise. These medications, prescribed and monitored by her healthcare team, can be a valuable tool in your weight loss arsenal.

The Role of Healthcare Providers

Dr. Hilda emphasizes the importance of working with experienced healthcare providers to achieve optimal results. Incorporating GLP-1 into your weight loss plan should always be done under the supervision of a medical professional. Regular check-ups and consultations ensure that your progress is monitored, and any potential side effects are managed effectively. Your healthcare team will tailor the use of GLP-1 to your individual needs, maximizing its benefits while minimizing risks. And when you are done losing weight, they will guide you on the maintenance program to ensure you never regain weight.

Behavior Modification: The Key to Lasting Change

The secret to long-term weight loss success lies in your mindset and habits. Dr. Hilda's behavior modification strategies will help you identify and change the behaviors that have been holding you back. Learn how to set realistic goals, manage stress, and stay motivated on your weight loss journey. By understanding and addressing the psychological aspects of weight loss, you'll be better equipped to maintain your progress and avoid the pitfalls of yo-yo dieting.

The Benefits of Following "The Ultimate Guide to lasting Weight loss."

By committing to the recommended guidelines, you will experience a multitude of benefits such as:

> **Improved Health:** Lower your risk of chronic diseases such as diabetes, heart disease, and hypertension.

> **Increased Energy:** Feel more vibrant and capable of tackling daily tasks with ease.

> **Enhanced Mood:** Experience the mental health benefits of regular exercise and a nutritious diet.

> **Sustainable Weight Loss:** Achieve and maintain a healthy weight without resorting to fad diets or extreme measures.

> **Boosted Confidence:** Feel proud of your accomplishments and enjoy a renewed sense of self-esteem.

> **Accelerated Weight Loss:** With the addition of GLP-1, achieve your weight loss goals faster than you ever thought possible.

> **Better Appetite Control:** GLP-1 helps you feel fuller longer, reducing the temptation to overeat.

> **Improved Blood Sugar Regulation:** Stabilize your blood sugar levels, lowering the risk of developing type 2 diabetes.

> **Professional Support:** Benefit from the guidance and supervision of healthcare professionals to ensure safe and effective use of GLP-1.

Take Action Today!

Are you ready to transform your life and achieve lasting weight loss success? Don't wait another day to start your journey. "The Ultimate Guide to lasting Weight loss" is your comprehensive guide to a healthier, happier you. Embrace the power of a balanced diet, regular exercise, and behavior modification, and watch as your goals become reality. With the added advantage of GLP-1 under Dr. Hilda and her healthcare team's guidance, you'll find yourself reaching your weight loss milestones sooner than you imagined. This hormone, combined with the strategies outlined in this guide, offers a powerful, science-backed approach to shedding pounds and maintaining a healthy weight for life.

Take the first step towards a brighter, healthier future. You have the power to change your life—let Dr. Hilda and her expert team guide you every step of the way. Together, we can make your weight loss dreams come true!

The journey to a healthier
you starts with a single step.
Make today the day you take that
step and never look back.

How the Program Works

Four Phases of the Dietary Program

The dietary program is divided into four distinct phases: the Detox Phase, the Modified Ketogenic Phase, the **Regular Phase**, and the Maintenance Phase. Each phase plays a crucial role in ensuring long-term success. The Detox Phase helps cleanse your body of toxins and prepares you for the journey ahead. The Modified Ketogenic Phase accelerates fat loss by shifting your body into a state of ketosis. The Regular Phase introduces a balanced diet that supports continued weight loss and overall health. Finally, the Maintenance Phase focuses on sustaining your weight loss and adopting lifelong healthy eating habits.

Detox Phase (Week 1)

The **Detox Phase** is the initial step in your weight loss journey. This phase focuses on cleansing your body of toxins and resetting your metabolism. By eliminating processed foods, sugars, and unhealthy fats, you prepare your body for effective weight loss. The Detox Phase typically lasts for one week and includes a diet rich in fruits, vegetables, lean proteins, and plenty of water. This phase helps reduce bloating, improve digestion, and increase energy levels, setting a solid foundation for the following phases.

Modified Ketogenic Phase (Week 2)

The **Modified Ketogenic Phase (Week 2)** is designed to accelerate fat loss by shifting your body into a state of ketosis, where it burns fat for fuel instead of carbohydrates. This phase involves a low-carb, high-fat diet that includes healthy fats like avocados, nuts, and olive oil, along with moderate protein intake. By drastically reducing carbohydrate intake, your body begins to utilize stored fat for energy, resulting in rapid weight loss. This phase lasts for 4 days, depending on your individual progress and goals.

Regular Phase
(Week 3 until you lose all the weight)

The Regular Phase introduces a more balanced diet while continuing to support weight loss. This phase reintroduces healthy carbohydrates, such as whole grains, fruits, and vegetables, in moderation. The focus is on maintaining a well-rounded diet that includes a variety of nutrients to support overall health. The Regular Phase helps stabilize your metabolism and ensures that weight loss continues at a steady pace. This phase is crucial for transitioning from a Modified ketogenic diet to a sustainable, long-term eating plan.

Maintenance Phase

The Maintenance Phase is the final step in the dietary program, aimed at sustaining your weight loss and adopting lifelong healthy eating habits. During this phase, you continue to follow a balanced diet while allowing for occasional indulgences. The key is to maintain portion control and make mindful food choices. The Maintenance Phase emphasizes consistency and moderation, helping you keep the weight off for good. This phase is ongoing and becomes a natural part of your lifestyle, ensuring lasting success.

Detox Phase (Week 1)

Why you need Detoxification

Detoxification is crucial to losing weight because we are currently exposed to daily stress, environmental toxins, and food additives. The body's metabolic process results in waste products that need to be removed from the body. Cleansing and detoxification of the body promotes good health and general wellbeing.

The liver is a major organ for detoxification, and it is the body's filtration system that filters out toxins from the body. It is like an oil filter in your car. The liver breaks down fats, carbohydrates, chemicals, and protein that we either eat or are exposed to daily. So, when excessive quantities of soda, fatty foods, etc. are consumed; it causes a lot of stress on the liver, making it almost impossible to burn fat and lose weight.

According to research, anyone who has been on a Standard American diet for more than two years would need periodic cleansing. Toxins can cause a lot of sluggish and digestive issues. It can cause your metabolism to slow down, your energy level to drop leading to the inability to burn stored fat, whether through exercise or diet.

Therefore, it is very important that you jump-start your weight loss program by detoxifying your major organs: the liver, colon, and kidneys. It will improve your digestive system, enhance metabolism, start burning stored fat, and help maintain a healthier and more beautiful you.

Follow the detoxification eating plan as strictly as possible to be able to achieve results and get your body into the fat burning mode. Every day for this one-week period:

> Drink 1 tablespoon of lemon juice first thing in the morning. This helps support the immune system and it also contracts the liver.

> Have 1 tablespoon of apple cider vinegar during the day. This helps to balance the pH of the body, eliminating waste acids, providing potassium and helps reduce water retention.

> Drink half your body weight in ounces of water. For instance, if you weigh 160 lbs., you need to drink at least 80 ounces of water daily.

> Eat at least two servings (the size of the palm of your hand) of very lean or lean protein (lean skinless chicken, turkey, or fish).

> Avoid processed foods, sugar, artificial sweeteners, refined carbohydrates, alcohol, caffeine, and salt.

> Choose fruits and plenty of vegetables from the fruit and vegetables list.

> Take the detox supplement as recommended.

Smart Eating throughout the Program

Choose your protein from this list during the DETOX phase of your weight loss program. It is necessary to eat a minimum of 10-15 oz. of protein (70-105 grams) per day. Also, do not eat more than 100 grams of carbohydrates. This amount can vary. During your weight loss program, women are allowed to eat about 1000-1200 calories per day and men are allowed no more than 1500 calories daily. Follow the guidelines recommended by one of our esteemed healthcare providers as plans are individualized.

Protein List

For women, they can eat approximately 3-4 ounces of protein per meal while men can eat between 4-6 ounces. Remember, this can vary for each person or the extent of physical activities they engage in. Note that one serving from the list equals one oz.

You can choose to eat Chicken, Turkey, Flounder, Haddock, Salmon, Catfish, Oysters, Halibut, Trout, Tuna, Crab, Lobster, Scallops, Shrimp, Venison, Buffalo, Ostrich, Processed meats such as Hot dog with 1 gram or less fat per oz., Egg whites, Egg substitutes, 1% cottage cheese, or Cheese with 3 gm or less fat/oz and Soft Tofu.

Trim visible excess fat and skin from meat and poultry. Bake, broil, boil or sauté in vegetable oil or butter. Avoid or eat sparingly highly pro-cessed meats like sausage, bacon and corned beef. Do not use lard, hydrogenated fats and avoid using bread crumbs or flour to prepare your protein.

> **Eat Beef, Pork, Veal or Lamb ONLY once a week.**

AVERAGE COUNT OF CALORIES PER OUNCE OF PROTEIN SOURCE	
Lean Meat	60 calories/ounce
Poultry	40 calories/ounce
Beef	70-80 calories
Lamb	70-80 calories
Pork	70-80 calories
Fish and seafood	30 calories/ounce
Eggs	80 calories
Cottage cheese	120 calories per ½ cup

***** Fruits & Vegetables List for Detox Phase ONLY *****

Eat raw, if possible, but if you would like to prepare foods - Steam or sauté' vegetables in a little vegetable broth- grill or boil

You are allowed to eat up to 4 servings from the list below. ½ cup of cooked vegetables equals one serving.

Fruits List

Apples, Apricot, Banana, Blackberries, Blueberries, Boysenberries, Cantaloupe, Cherries (12), Dates, fresh Figs, fresh, Fresh fruit cup, Fruit cocktail (no sugar added), Pineapple, Plums, Raisins, Strawberries, Grapefruit, Grapes, Guava, Honeydew melon, Kiwi fruit, Kumquats, Lemon, Lychees, Mandarin, Orange, Mango, Nectarine, Nectars, Papaya, Passion fruit, Peach, Pear, Pomegranate, Prunes, Raspberries.

Vegetables List

Alfalfa Sprouts, Artichokes, Asparagus, Bean sprouts, Bell pepper, Bok Choy, Broccoli, Brussels sprouts, Cabbage, Cauliflower, Celery, Chard, Collard greens, Cucumber, Eggplant, Green beans, Hot peppers, Jicama, Kale, Leeks, Lettuce (all types), Mushrooms, Okra, Olives, Onions, Parsley, Radishes, Sauerkraut (no sugar added), Snow peas, Spaghetti squash, Spinach, Tomatoes, Watercress, Water chestnuts, Yellow squash, Zucchini.

Modified Ketogenic Phase [Week 2]

The Modified Ketogenic Phase is designed to accelerate fat loss by shifting your body into a state of ketosis, where it burns fat for fuel instead of carbohydrates.

This phase involves a low-carb, high-fat diet that includes healthy fats like avocados, nuts, and olive oil, along with moderate protein intake. By drastically reducing carbohydrate intake, your body begins to utilize stored fat for energy, resulting in rapid weight loss. This phase lasts for 4 days only and can be repeated throughout the program and especially when you feel you have plateaued depending on your individual progress and goals.

Note that Caffeine and alcohol can affect ketosis and fat burning.

The goal of the first 4 days of your eating plan in the 2nd week is to eat protein ONLY to induce KETOSIS. This means your body will start burning fatty tissue and stored carbohydrates will be depleted. Ketosis is achieved by consuming a diet that consists of protein only. You must avoid any form of carbohydrate.

Regular Phase (From day 5 in the 2nd week)

The Regular Phase introduces a more balanced diet while continuing to support weight loss. This phase reintroduces healthy carbohydrates, such as whole grains, fruits, and vegetables, in moderation. The focus is on maintaining a well-rounded diet that includes a variety of nutrients to support overall health. The Regular Phase helps stabilize your metabolism and ensures that weight loss continues at a steady pace. This phase is crucial for transitioning from a Modified ketogenic diet to a sustainable, long-term eating plan.

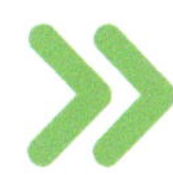

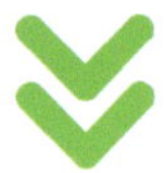

On day 5, reintroduce fruits and vegetables to your diet from this recommend list below.

2 FRUIT SERVINGS PER DAY	
Apples	1 medium
Blueberries	¼ cup
Cherries	12 large
Grapefruit	½ cup
Grapes	12
Guava	1 small
Orange	1 medium
Peach	1 medium
Strawberries	6
Raspberries	6
Blackberries	6

2 VEGETABLE SERVINGS PER DAY
Artichokes
Asparagus
Bamboo Shoots
Broccoli
Beans (green, yellow)
Brussels Sprouts
Cabbage
Cauliflower
Celery, celery leaves
Greens (collard)
Cucumber
Eggplant
Mushrooms
Peppers (green, red, sweet, hot)
Sauerkraut (no sugar added)
Spinach
Onions
Radish

Remember: Your choices of fruits and vegetables are going to dictate the rate of your weight loss. We recommend sticking to eating mostly these fruits and vegetables till you reach your goal weight.

Nourish your body with the right foods, and it will reward you with energy, vitality, and longevity. Your plate is your power.

Other Dietary Recommendations

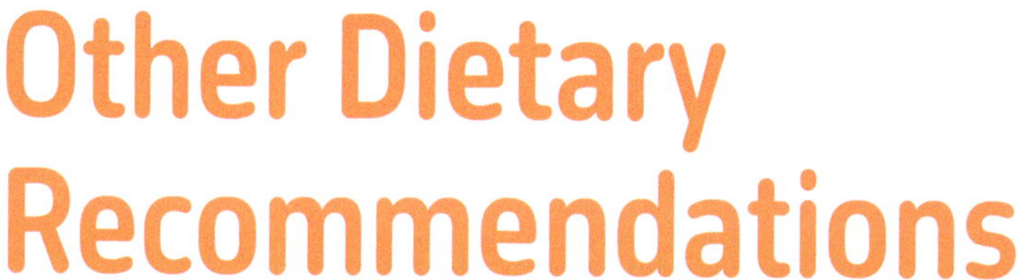

DO NOT EAT- Beets, bread, carrots, pasta, rice, tomatoes or lima beans.

Avoid eating starchy vegetables such as potatoes, yam, peas, corn, or winter squash. They are not allowed in your diet.

Protein Shakes:
Make sure it has no more than 3 grams of sugar.

Free selections:
Butter buds, salt, pepper, seasonings, spices, dry barbecue spices, fat free broth, white and red wine vinegar, Tabasco hot sauce, lemon and lime juice, mustard, miracle whip free, cocktail sauce, ½ cup of diet gelatin, lettuce (all types), Braggs Liquid Amino (which can be used on your salad, fish, chicken or vegetables).

Sugar Products:
Instead of sugar products, you may use Stevia, Trivia, zero sugar or Cinnamon. These are all natural sweeteners with zero calories, and they can be added to your coffee, tea or on any fruit.

Avoid sugars, corn-syrup or high sodium condiments.

Beverages and Fluids:
Calorie free flavored water, decaf diet sodas, decaf coffee and tea, regular coffee (limit to 1 cup), crystal light, sugar free country time lemonade, diet seltzer, diet mineral water, any calorie free- caffeine, diet free drinks. Limit Milk, Juices or Creamers.

Salad Dressing:
2 tbsp low fat or fat free dressing with no more than 30 calories per tbsp. Also, may use 1 tbsp olive oil and red vinegar (free selection), Balsamic vinegarette dressing. Check out other healthy salad dressings in the appendix section).

Daily fluid requirements:
1 gallon (128 oz./16-8oz glasses) of fluids; 64 ounces must come from water.

Healthy Nuts and Seeds

Incorporating nuts and seeds into your diet can provide essential nutrients and healthy fats that support weight loss. Here are some healthy options along with recommended portion sizes:

Almonds-1 ounce (about 23 almonds), Walnuts-1 ounce (about 14 halves), Pistachios- 1 ounce (about 49 pistachios), Chia Seeds-1 tablespoon, Flaxseeds-1 tablespoon (ground), Sunflower Seeds- 1 ounce (about 3 tablespoons), Pumpkin Seeds-1 ounce (about 2 tablespoons)

Tips for Including Nuts and Seeds in Your Diet

> **Portion Control:** Nuts and seeds are calorie-dense, so it's important to stick to recommended serving sizes to avoid overconsumption.

> **Snacking:** Use nuts and seeds as a healthy snack alternative to chips or candy.

> **Salads and Yogurt:** Add a tablespoon of chia seeds or a handful of nuts to salads, yogurt, or oatmeal for added crunch and nutrients.

> **Smoothies:** Blend ground flaxseeds or chia seeds into smoothies for an extra nutritional boost.

> **Baking:** Incorporate nuts and seeds into homemade granola bars or muffins.

By incorporating these healthy nuts and seeds in moderation, you can enjoy their nutritional benefits while supporting your weight loss goals.

Portion Size Guide

For each meal, here's a general guide:

> High protein foods such as Meat, Fish, Poultry, and beans should be served in quantities the size of a palm for women and two palm-sized servings for men.

> Salads and Vegetables: Two servings the size of fists for males and one for women

> High-Carbohydrate foods such as Whole grains and starchy vegetables, one cupped-hand quantity for women and two for men

> High-fat foods: nuts, butter, and oils; one thumb-sized serving for women, two for men.

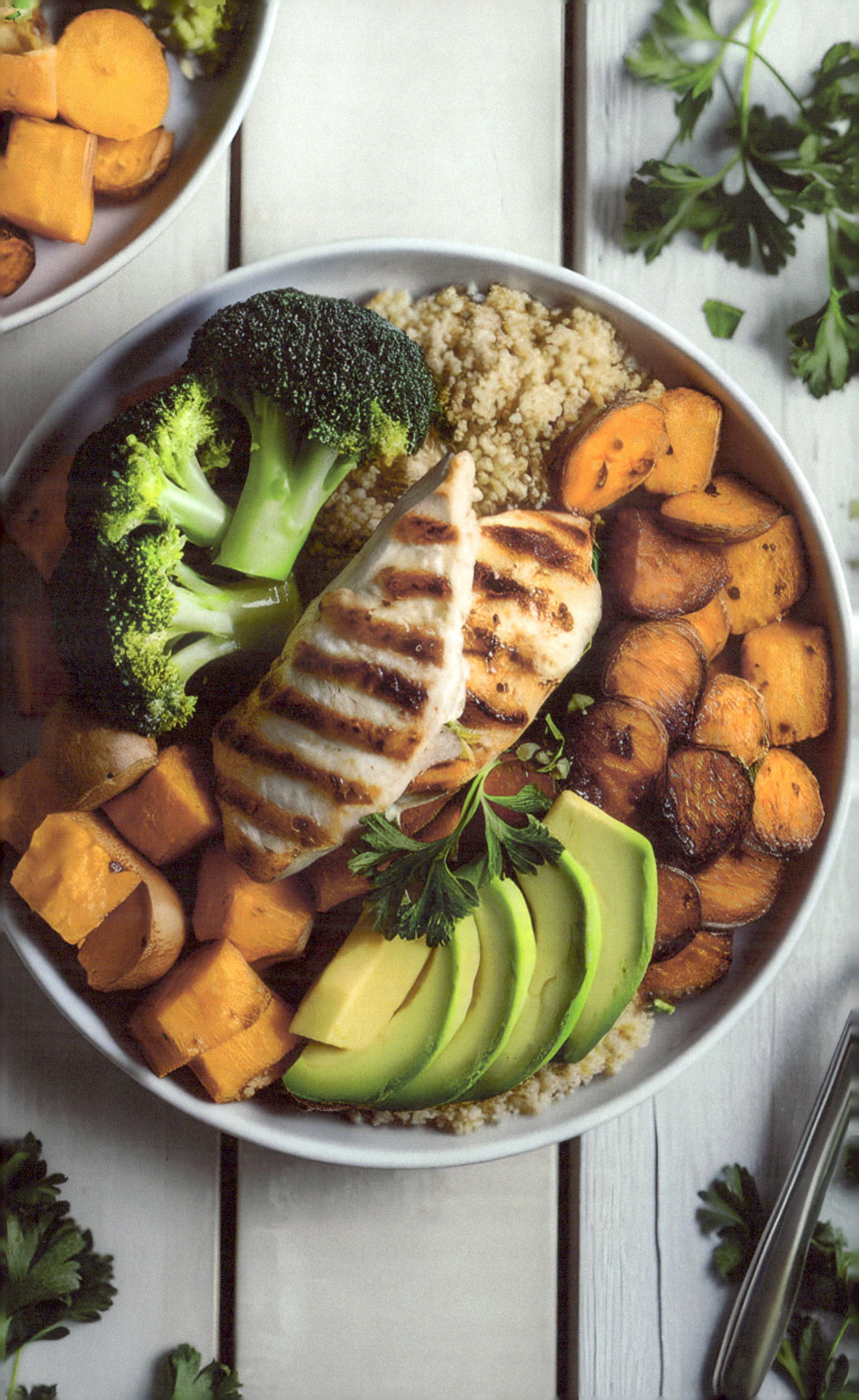

Why you need to Stay well Hydrated

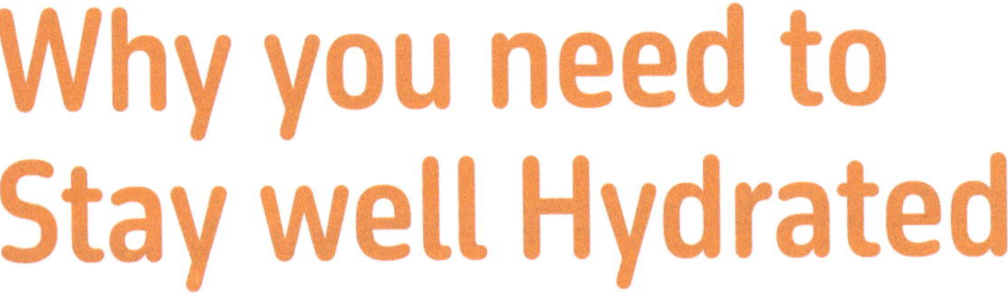

Drinking plenty of water and staying well hydrated is crucial for effective weight loss and overall health. Here's why staying hydrated plays a significant role in your weight loss journey:

> **Enhances Metabolism:** Drinking water can temporarily boost your metabolism. Studies have shown that drinking 500 ml of water can increase resting energy expenditure by 24–30% for about an hour. This boost in metabolism helps burn more calories throughout the day.

> **Suppresses Appetite:** Sometimes, thirst is mistaken for hunger. Drinking water before meals can help you feel fuller, leading to reduced calorie intake. A study found that people who drank 500 ml of water before meals ate fewer calories and lost 44% more weight over 12 weeks compared to those who didn't.

> **Aids Digestion:** Proper hydration is essential for healthy digestion. Water helps break down food, allowing your body to absorb nutrients effectively. It also prevents constipation, which can cause bloating and discomfort.

> **Supports Exercise Performance:** Staying hydrated is crucial for optimal physical performance. Dehydration can lead to reduced strength, endurance, and performance, making it harder to stick to your exercise routine and burn calories.

> **Boosts Fat Burning:** Water is involved in the process of lipolysis, the breakdown of fat in the body. The first step of lipolysis is hydrolysis, which requires water. Adequate hydration supports the body's ability to burn fat for energy.

> **Reduces Liquid Calorie Intake:** Choosing water over sugary beverages like sodas, juices, or energy drinks can significantly reduce your calorie intake. These beverages are often high in empty calories and can contribute to weight gain.

> **Improves Mood and Energy Levels:** Dehydration can lead to fatigue, irritability, and reduced cognitive function. Drinking enough water helps

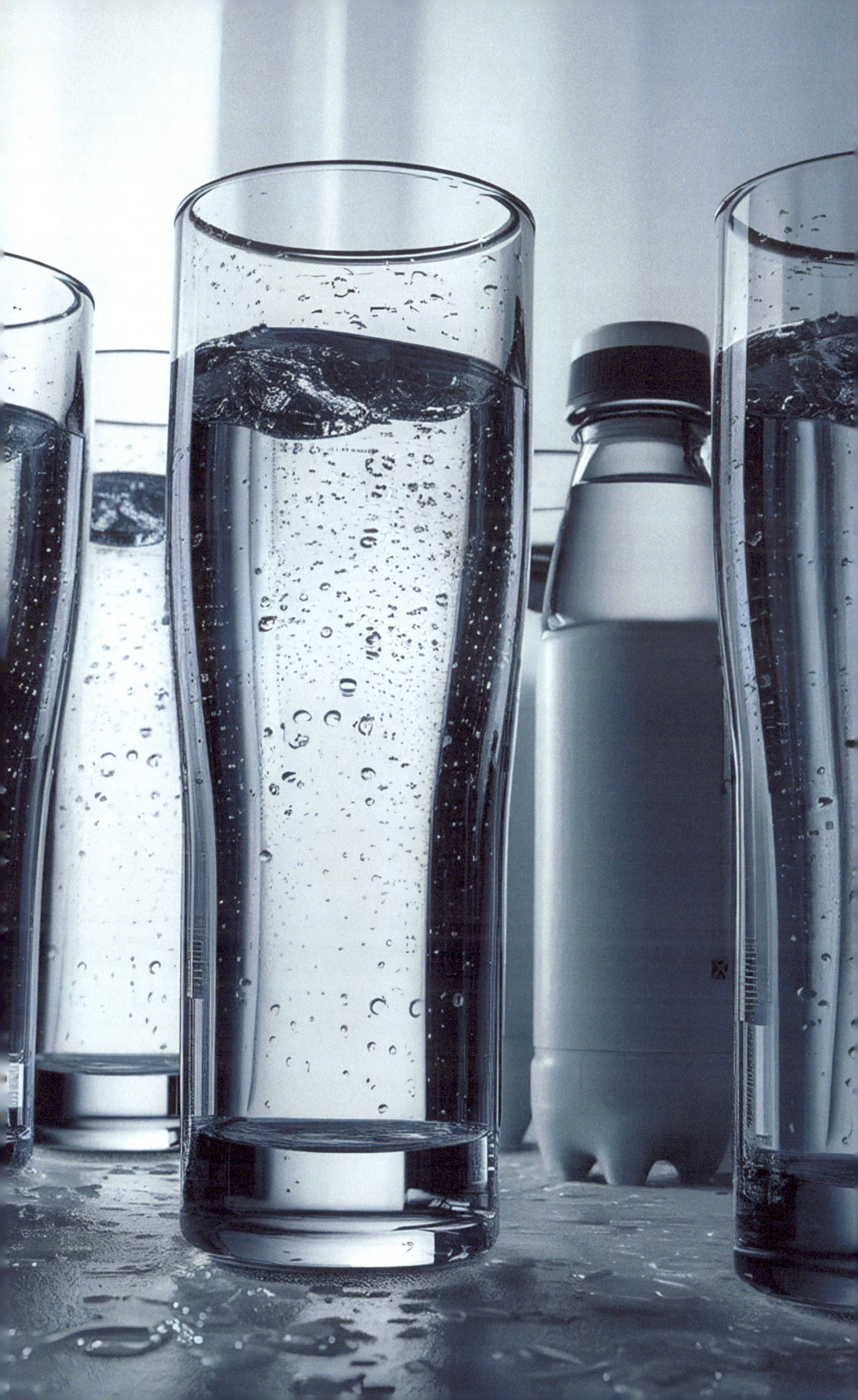

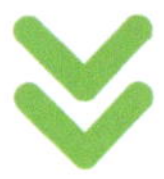

maintain energy levels and mood, making it easier to stay motivated and focused on your weight loss goals.

> **Helps Detoxify the Body:** Water aids in flushing out toxins and waste products through urine and sweat. This detoxification process is essential for maintaining overall health and can support weight loss efforts.

> **Promotes Healthy Skin:** Proper hydration keeps your skin healthy and glowing. As you lose weight, drinking water can help your skin remain elastic and firm, reducing the appearance of sagging or loose skin.

> **Regulates Body Temperature:** Water helps regulate body temperature, especially during physical activity. Staying hydrated prevents overheating and ensures your body functions optimally during workouts.

Tips for Staying well Hydrated

> **Carry a Water Bottle:** Keep a water bottle with you throughout the day to remind yourself to drink water regularly.

> **Set Reminders:** Use phone apps or alarms to remind you to drink water at regular intervals.

> **Flavor Your Water:** If plain water is too boring, add slices of fruit, cucumber, or mint to enhance the flavor without adding calories.

> **Drink Before Meals:** Have a glass of water before each meal to help control your appetite.

> **Monitor Your Intake:** Aim for at least 8-10 glasses of water per day, but adjust based on your activity level, climate, and individual needs.

> **Eat Water-Rich Foods:** Include fruits and vegetables with high water content in your diet, such as cucumbers and oranges.

Drinking enough water is a simple yet powerful tool in your weight loss arsenal. By enhancing metabolism, suppressing appetite, aiding digestion, and supporting exercise performance, proper hydration plays a pivotal role in achieving and maintaining a healthy weight. Make hydration a priority, and you'll be better equipped to reach your weight loss goals while enjoying improved overall health and well-being.

The Importance of Limiting Sugar and Salt in your Diet

Limiting sugar and salt in your diet is crucial for maintaining overall health and well-being. Excessive intake of sugar and salt is linked to a range of serious health issues, making it important to be mindful of how much you consume.

Negative Impact on Health

Sugar: Consuming too much sugar can lead to a variety of health problems. It's a major contributor to obesity, as sugary foods and drinks are often high in calories but low in nutritional value. Over time, high sugar intake can lead to insulin resistance, increasing the risk of type 2 diabetes. It also promotes tooth decay and can contribute to heart disease by raising levels of harmful cholesterol and triglycerides in the blood.

Salt: Excessive salt intake is primarily associated with high blood pressure (hypertension), a major risk factor for heart disease and stroke. High salt levels can also cause your body to retain water, leading to bloating and swelling. Over time, too much salt can strain your kidneys and lead to kidney disease, and it may also contribute to osteoporosis by causing calcium loss from bones.

Potassium-rich foods play a crucial role in maintaining healthy blood pressure by helping to balance the effects of sodium in your body. When you consume enough potassium, it helps relax blood vessel walls and excrete excess sodium through urine, which can lower blood pressure and reduce the risk of heart disease. Additionally, potassium helps prevent muscle cramps by ensuring proper muscle function
and fluid balance, making it an essential nutrient for those who are active or prone to cramping. Foods like bananas, sweet potatoes, plantains, broccoli, spinach, and avocados are excellent sources of potassium and can contribute to overall cardiovascular and muscular health.

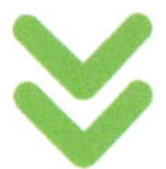

Different Names for Sugar and Salt

Sugar comes in many forms and can be hidden in processed foods under various names. Some common names for sugar include:

> Sucrose

> Fructose

> Glucose

> High fructose corn syrup (HFCS)

> Cane sugar

> Molasses

> Honey

> Agave nectar

> Maltose

> Dextrose

Salt can also be listed under different names, especially in processed foods. These include:

> Sodium chloride (table salt)

> Sodium bicarbonate (baking soda)

> Monosodium glutamate (MSG)

> Sodium nitrate/nitrite

> Disodium phosphate

> Sodium alginate

Healthy Alternatives

Instead of relying on sugar and salt to enhance flavor, consider these healthier alternatives:

For Sugar:

> **Stevia:** A natural sweetener derived from the leaves of the Stevia plant. It has no calories and does not raise blood sugar levels.

> **Monk Fruit:** Another natural sweetener, monk fruit extract is low in calories and much sweeter than sugar.

> **Honey or Maple Syrup:** While still a form of sugar, these options are less processed and contain some nutrients. Use them sparingly.

❯ **Cinnamon or Vanilla Extract:** These can add sweetness without the added sugar, making them great for flavoring foods like oatmeal or coffee.

For Salt:

❯ **Herbs and Spices:** Garlic, basil, oregano, cumin, and other herbs and spices can add a depth of flavor without the need for salt.

❯ **Lemon Juice or Vinegar:** These acidic options can enhance the flavor of food and reduce the need for added salt.

❯ **Potassium Chloride:** A salt substitute that tastes similar to table salt but is lower in sodium. However, consult with a healthcare provider before using this, especially if you have kidney issues.

❯ **Nutritional Yeast:** A cheesy-flavored seasoning that's low in sodium and rich in nutrients like B vitamins.

By being aware of the hidden sources of sugar and salt and choosing healthier alternatives, you can significantly reduce your risk of chronic diseases and improve your overall health.

How to read a Food Label

Understanding how to read food labels is essential for making healthier choices when you're shopping. Look for a food label on packaged foods. It can help you make good food choices.

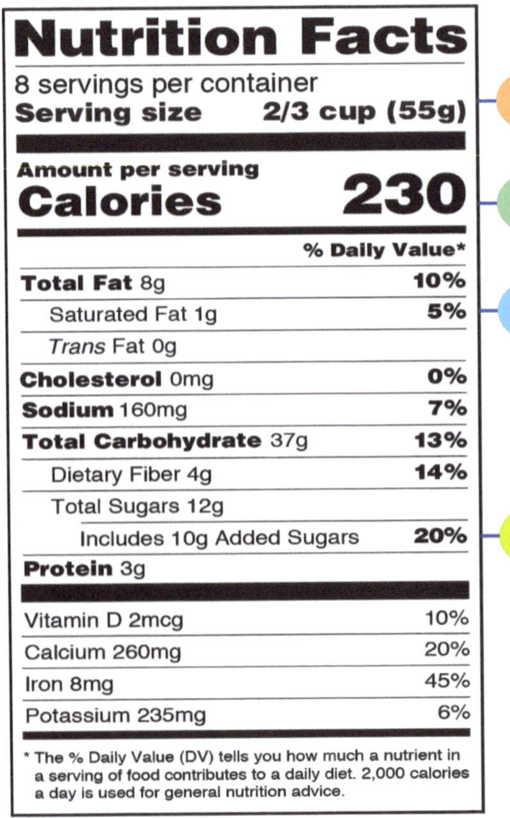

Nutrition Facts	
8 servings per container	
Serving size	**2/3 cup (55g)**
Amount per serving	
Calories	**230**
	% Daily Value*
Total Fat 8g	**10%**
Saturated Fat 1g	**5%**
Trans Fat 0g	
Cholesterol 0mg	**0%**
Sodium 160mg	**7%**
Total Carbohydrate 37g	**13%**
Dietary Fiber 4g	**14%**
Total Sugars 12g	
Includes 10g Added Sugars	**20%**
Protein 3g	
Vitamin D 2mcg	10%
Calcium 260mg	20%
Iron 8mg	45%
Potassium 235mg	6%

* The % Daily Value (DV) tells you how much a nutrient in a serving of food contributes to a daily diet. 2,000 calories a day is used for general nutrition advice.

1. Serving size shows a realistic amount of the food. Similar types of food have similar serving sizes.

2. Calories from fat can help you decide if a food has too much fat.

3. List of nutrients can help you decide if a food has too much fat.

4. % Daily value shows how the food fits into your overall diet.

Food labels provide important information about the nutritional content of a product, helping you determine if it fits into your diet and health goals. Here's a guide to help you navigate food labels:

1. Start with the Serving Size

The serving size is listed at the top of the label and tells you the amount of food the nutritional information applies to. All the other numbers on the label are based on this serving size. Pay attention to this because it's easy to consume more than the serving size, which means you'll need to adjust the nutritional values accordingly.

2. Check the Calories

Calories indicate how much energy you'll get from a serving of the food. If you're trying to manage your weight, knowing the calorie content is crucial. Remember, if you eat more than one serving, you'll need to multiply the calories by the number of servings you consume.

3. Look at the Nutrients to Limit

❯ Total Fat, Saturated Fat, and Trans Fat: High levels of these fats, especially trans fats, are linked to heart disease. Aim for products with low amounts of saturated fat and avoid trans fats whenever possible.

❯ Cholesterol: High cholesterol intake can contribute to heart disease, so it's best to keep this low.

❯ Sodium (Salt): Too much sodium can lead to high blood pressure, so look for products that are low in sodium.

❯ Sugars: The label will list both natural and added sugars. Added sugars are the ones you want to limit, as they contribute to weight gain and other health issues.

4. Focus on Nutrients You Need More Of

❯ Dietary Fiber: Fiber is important for digestive health and can help you feel full, which may aid in weight management. Look for foods with higher fiber content.

❯ Vitamins and Minerals: The label may include nutrients like Vitamin D, Calcium, Iron, and Potassium, which are essential for maintaining good health. Aim to choose foods that are high in these nutrients.

5. Understand the Percent Daily Value (%DV)

The % Daily Value on a label shows you how much of a nutrient is in one serving of food, compared to how much you should consume in a day (based on a 2,000-calorie diet).

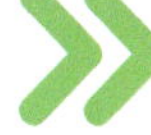

> 5% DV or less is considered low for nutrients, so it's good for things like fat, cholesterol, and sodium.

> 20% DV or more is considered high, which is good for nutrients you want more of, like fiber, vitamins, and minerals.

6. Identify Ingredients

The ingredients list is usually found below the Nutrition Facts panel. Ingredients are listed in order of quantity, from highest to lowest.

> Watch out for hidden sugars: Ingredients like high-fructose corn syrup, cane sugar, and fruit juice concentrate are all forms of added sugars.

> Limit artificial additives: Ingredients like artificial colors, flavors, and preservatives may be best avoided, especially if you're aiming for a more natural diet.

7. Be Aware of Claims

Food packaging often features health claims like "low fat," "reduced sodium," or "high in fiber." While these can be helpful, they can also be misleading. Always check the Nutrition Facts label to verify the claims. For example:

> "Low fat" doesn't necessarily mean low calories; the product might have added sugars.

> "Natural" is not regulated by the FDA, so it doesn't guarantee the product is healthy.

8. Consider the Whole Product

Don't just focus on one aspect of the label, like calories or sugar content. Consider the whole product and how it fits into your overall diet. For example, a product might be low in calories but high in sodium or lacking in essential nutrients.

9. Check for Allergens

If you have food allergies, it's crucial to read the label for allergen information. Common allergens like nuts, dairy, and gluten are usually highlighted at the end of the ingredients list.

By taking the time to read and understand food labels, you can make informed decisions that support your health and wellness goals.

Averting High Cholesterol

Averting high cholesterol is essential for maintaining heart health and reducing the risk of cardiovascular diseases. Elevated cholesterol levels can lead to the buildup of plaque in arteries, increasing the risk of heart attacks and strokes.

One of the most effective ways to manage cholesterol is by making healthier food choices and preparing meals in ways that promote heart health. Opt for cooking methods like grilling, baking, steaming, and poaching instead of frying, which can add unhealthy fats to your diet. Incorporating more fruits, vegetables, whole grains, and lean proteins into your meals can significantly lower cholesterol levels.

Using herbs and spices instead of salt to flavor dishes can enhance taste without raising cholesterol. Replacing saturated and trans fats with healthier fats, such as those found in olive oil, avocados, and nuts, can improve your lipid profile. Regular consumption of fatty fish rich in omega-3 fatty acids, like salmon and mackerel, also supports healthy cholesterol levels. Reading nutrition labels and choosing foods low in cholesterol and high in fiber can further aid in cholesterol management. By adopting these meal preparation practices and dietary changes, you can effectively manage and reduce cholesterol levels, promoting overall heart health.

SOURCE OF FAT OR CHOLESTEROL	TRY INSTEAD
Fried foods	Steaming, boiling, or baking vegetables. Broiling, roasting, or baking meat on a rack so fat drain off.
Using butter and margarine for flavor	Herbs and spices
Salad dressing	Lemon juice or vinegar
Butter and shortening baking	Margarine or oil
Whole milk	Skim milk
Sour cream and mayonnaise	Plain low-fat yogurt
Fatty cuts of meat	Leaner cuts of meat; trim fat
Egg yolks or more whites than yolk	Using just the whites
Chicken skin	Removing skin before cooking

Incorporating Physical Activities

The best way to accelerate and maintain your weight loss is to incorporate physical activities or some form of a moderate exercise program.

Strenuous exercises that may lead to injury must be avoided. Over exercising may cause more harm than good. The goal of our program is to balance your food intake and balance your exercise program. Excessive exercise is essential in decreasing insulin resistance, which causes a decrease in body fat. This fat reduction will make you healthier and decrease your chances of getting diabetes, hypertensions, stroke, and other chronic illnesses.

Benefits of exercise:

> Manage your weight
> Strengthen your cardiovascular and respiratory system
> Keep muscles and bones strong
> Ease depression and help manage pain and stress
> Prevent and manage diabetes
> Reduce the risk of certain types of cancer
> Sleep better

Aerobic exercise:

Our program encourages aerobic exercise up to 6 days a week. The intensity should be moderate since intense aerobic exercise will decrease the use of fat as energy since the muscles will derive their energy from glucose rather than fat.

The following are forms of aerobic activities:

> Running
> Walking
> Biking
> Elliptical
> Swimming

Strength Training

The body can synthesize muscle mass at any age and maintaining muscle mass will increase your immune function as you age. Strength training will increase muscle fibers and the amino acid glutamine is stored in the muscle fibers. Glutamine is essential for your immune function and thus maintaining muscle mass will assure that there is adequate amount of this amino acid when the body requires it in a crisis. Muscle mass also aids the body in extracting glucose from the bloodstream and causing a drop in the insulin requirements. Our program recommends strength training 3 days a week.

UPPER BODY ROUTINES	LOWER BODY ROUTINES
Chess press	Narrow Squats
Shoulder press	Wide Squat
Bicep's curl	Forward and Backward Lunges
Triceps dip	Straight leg rise
Lateral and front rise	Easy up abdominal sit up

The following exercises should be done on alternate days and the goal is to eventually do 3 sets of each exercise with 12 repetitions in each set.

Stretching

Rules of stretching

> Lengthen the body throughout each movement
> Do not bounce, pull, or force a stretch

Stretches

> Side stretch
> Chest and shoulder stretch
> Hamstrings stretch
> Triceps stretch
> Biceps stretch
> Back stretch
> Quadriceps stretch
> Glutes stretch

Stretching should be done 3 days a week when not strength training.

Sample Weekly Exercises

DAY 1	DAY 2	DAY 3	DAY 4	DAY 5	DAY 6
Aerobic 10 min.	Aerobic 10 min.	Aerobic 10 min.	Aerobic 10 min.	Aerobic 10 min.	Aerobic 10 min.
Strength Training 1. chest press 2. shoulder press 3. lateral and front rise 10 min	Stretching 10 min.	Stretching Training 1. biceps curl 2. triceps curl 3. forward lunge 10 min.	Stretching 10 min.	Stretching Training 1. narrow squat 2. Wide squat 10 min.	Stretching 10 min.
Aerobic 10 min.	Aerobic 10 min.	Aerobic 10 min.	Aerobic 10 min.	Aerobic 10 min.	Aerobic 10 min.

Note: Abdominal exercises should be performed during each session using the easy up abdominal sit up. There should be a day of rest, preferably in the middle of the week.

The duration and intensity of the program can be increased as you become better conditioned but remember that intense exercise can cause more harm than good.

Chair Exercises for Added Strength

Chair exercises are an excellent way to build strength, especially for individuals who may have limited mobility, are recovering from an injury, or simply prefer a seated workout. These exercises can be performed at home, using a sturdy chair with no wheels. Here are some effective chair exercises that can help build strength:

1. Seated Leg Lifts

▶ **How to Perform:** Sit tall in the chair with your feet flat on the floor. Extend one leg straight out in front of you, keeping it as straight as possible without locking your knee. Hold for a few seconds, then lower the leg without letting your foot touch the floor. Repeat for 10-15 reps on each leg.

▶ **Benefits:** This exercise strengthens the quadriceps and helps improve leg stability.

2. Chair Squats

▶ **How to Perform:** Stand in front of the chair with your feet shoulder-width apart. Lower yourself down as if you're going to sit, but just tap the chair with your glutes before standing back up. Use your arms for balance, but avoid using them to push off the chair. Repeat for 10-15 reps.

▶ **Benefits:** Chair squats target the thighs, hips, and glutes, building lower body strength and improving balance.

3. Seated Arm Curls

▶ **How to Perform:** Sit up straight with your back against the chair. Hold a dumbbell or water bottle in each hand with your arms by your sides. Slowly curl the weights up toward your shoulders, keeping your elbows close to your body. Lower the weights back down slowly. Perform 10-15 reps.

▶ **Benefits:** This exercise strengthens the biceps and improves upper arm tone.

4. Seated Marches

▶ **How to Perform:** Sit at the edge of the chair with your back straight and feet flat on the floor. Lift one knee as high as possible, mimicking

the motion of marching, then lower it back down. Alternate between legs for 20-30 seconds.

> **Benefits:** Seated marches work the hip flexors and lower abs, improving core strength and hip mobility.

5. Seated Chest Press

> **How to Perform:** Sit upright with a resistance band wrapped around the back of the chair. Hold the ends of the band in each hand, with your elbows bent and hands at chest level. Press your hands forward until your arms are fully extended, then slowly bring them back to the starting position. Perform 10-15 reps.

> **Benefits:** This exercise targets the chest, shoulders, and triceps, helping to build upper body strength.

6. Seated Knee Extensions

> **How to Perform:** Sit up straight with your back against the chair. Extend one leg straight out, keeping your foot flexed. Slowly lower the leg back down. Perform 10-15 reps on each leg.

> **Benefits:** This exercise strengthens the quadriceps and helps improve knee stability.

7. Chair Dips

> **How to Perform:** Sit on the edge of the chair with your hands gripping the front of the seat, fingers facing forward. Slide your butt off the chair, keeping your legs bent and feet flat on the floor. Lower your body by bending your elbows to about a 90-degree angle, then push back up. Perform 10-12 reps.

> **Benefits:** Chair dips strengthen the triceps, shoulders, and chest.

8. Seated Side Bends

> **How to Perform:** Sit up straight with your feet flat on the floor. Place one hand behind your head, and slowly lean to the opposite side, reaching toward the floor with your free hand. Return to the starting position and repeat on the other side. Perform 10 reps on each side.

> **Benefits:** This exercise strengthens the obliques and helps improve core stability.

Chair exercises are an excellent way to strengthen your muscles and improve flexibility and balance, all while staying comfortably seated. They are particularly beneficial for individuals with limited mobility or those looking for low-impact strength training options. Regular practice of these exercises can lead to improved overall fitness and greater independence in daily activities.

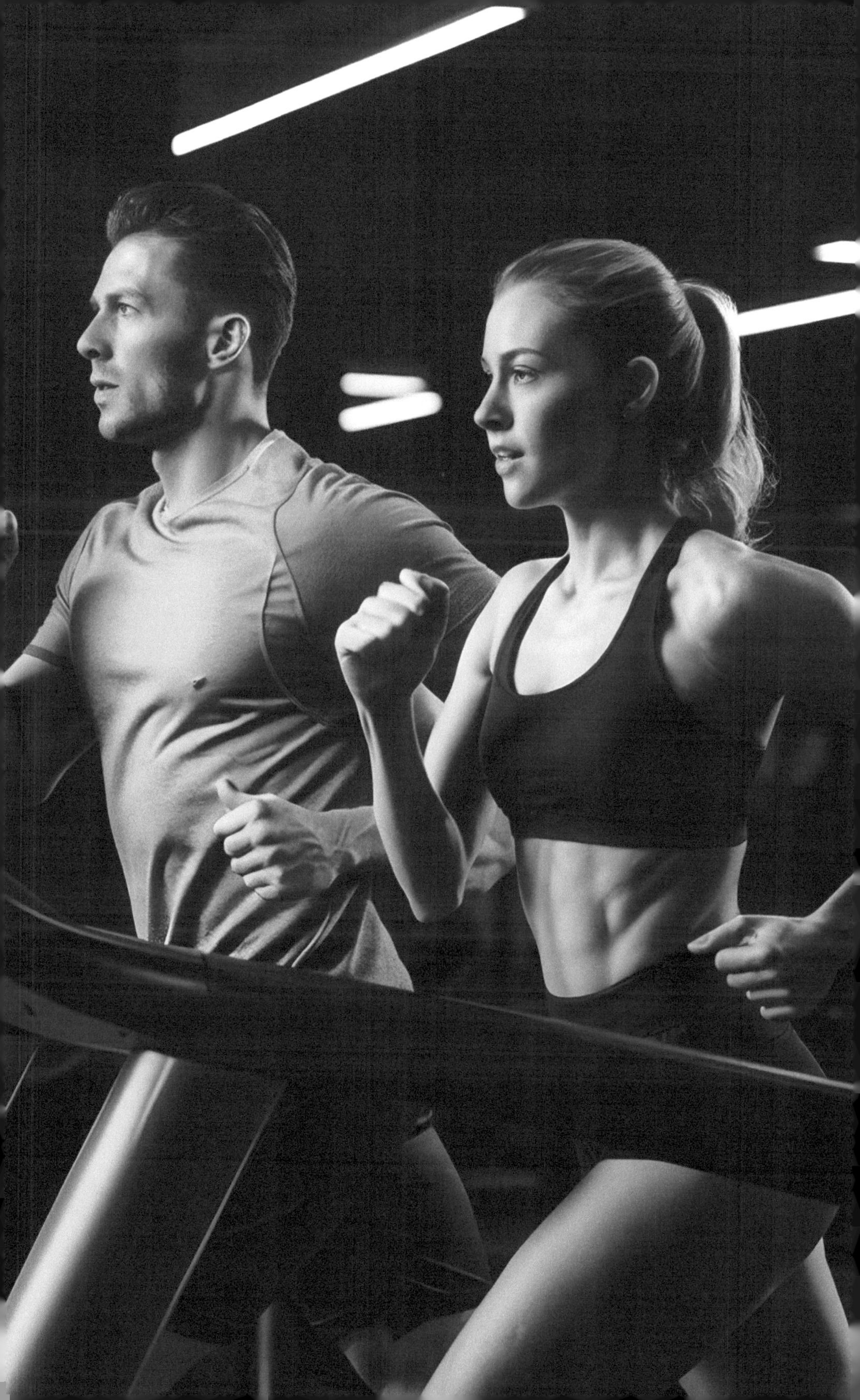

Exercise for the Larger bodied individual

For heavy individuals, starting an exercise routine can be challenging, but it is crucial for improving health and aiding weight loss. It's important to choose exercises that are low-impact and safe to minimize the risk of injury. These are some recommended exercises:

1. Walking

> Walking is a simple, low-impact exercise that can be done anywhere.

> Benefits: Improves cardiovascular health, burns calories, and enhances mood.

> Tips: Start with short distances and gradually increase the duration and pace. Aim for 10-15 minutes initially and work up to 30 minutes or more.

2. Swimming

> Swimming and water aerobics provide a full-body workout without putting stress on the joints.

> Benefits: Improves cardiovascular health, strengthens muscles, and increases flexibility.

> Tips: Start with basic swimming strokes or join a water aerobics class designed for beginners.

3. Chair Exercises

> Exercises performed while sitting in a chair, such as seated leg lifts, arm circles, and seated marches.

> Benefits: Improves muscle strength and flexibility without putting pressure on the joints.

> Tips: Use a sturdy chair without wheels and perform exercises slowly and deliberately.

4. Resistance Band Exercises

❯ Using resistance bands to perform exercises like bicep curls, seated rows, and leg presses.

❯ Benefits: Builds muscle strength, enhances flexibility, and can be done seated or standing.

❯ Tips: Choose a resistance band with appropriate resistance level and perform exercises in a controlled manner.

5. Recumbent Bike

❯ A stationary bike that allows you to sit in a reclined position while pedaling.

❯ Benefits: Low-impact cardiovascular exercise that strengthens the legs and improves endurance.

❯ Tips: Start with short sessions (10-15 minutes) and gradually increase the duration.

6. Tai Chi

❯ A gentle form of martial arts that involves slow, controlled movements and deep breathing.

❯ Benefits: Improves balance, flexibility, and mental well-being.

❯ Tips: Look for beginner classes or instructional videos to learn the basic movements.

7. Stretching

❯ Simple stretches that can be done seated or standing to improve flexibility and range of motion.

❯ Benefits: Enhances flexibility, reduces muscle tension, and prepares the body for other exercises.

❯ Tips: Hold each stretch for 20-30 seconds and avoid bouncing or jerking movements.

8. Bodyweight Exercises

❯ Exercises that use your body weight as resistance, such as wall push-ups, modified squats, and standing leg lifts.

❯ Benefits: Builds strength and endurance without the need for equipment.

> Tips: Perform exercises slowly and focus on maintaining proper form.

9. Water Walking

> Walking in shallow water, such as a pool, provides resistance and reduces stress on the joints.

> Benefits: Enhances cardiovascular health, improves muscle strength, and is easy on the joints.

> Tips: Start with short sessions and gradually increase the duration.

10. Dance

> Low-impact dance routines, such as Zumba Gold or beginner dance classes.

> Benefits: Increases cardiovascular health, improves coordination, and is a fun way to exercise.

> Tips: Choose routines designed for beginners or those with limited mobility.

Every step you take in your workout today is a stride toward a healthier, stronger tomorrow. Embrace the journey, one movement at a time.

Behavior Modification for Weight Management

Weight management involves adopting a healthy lifestyle that includes knowledge of nutrition and exercise, a positive attitude, and the right kind of motivation. Internal motives such as better health, increased energy, self-esteem, and personal control increase your chances of lifelong weight management success.

Remember to have realistic goals and think about long-term success. Believe in yourself and you can do it! The following information will give you ideas to help you meet your goals.

Control Your Home Environment:

> Eat only while sitting down at the kitchen or dining room table. Do not eat while watching television, reading, cooking, talking on the phone, standing at the refrigerator, or working on the computer. Keep tempting foods out of the house — do not buy them.

> Have low-calorie foods ready to eat. Unless you are preparing a meal, stay out of the kitchen. Have healthy snacks at your disposal, such as small pieces of fruit, vegetables, canned fruit, pretzels, low-fat string cheese and nonfat cottage cheese.

Control Your Work Environment:

> Do not eat at your desk or keep tempting snacks at your desk. If you get hungry between meals, plan healthy snacks, and bring them with you to work. During your breaks, go for a walk instead of eating. If you work around food, plan the one item you will eat at mealtime.

> Make it inconvenient to nibble on food by chewing gum, sugarless candy or drinking water or another low-calorie beverage. Do not work through meals. Skipping meals slows down metabolism and may result in overeating at the next meal.

> If food is available for special occasions, either pick the healthiest item, nibble on low-fat snacks brought from home, do not have anything offered, choose one option, and have a small amount, or have only one beverage.

Control Your Mealtime Environment:

> Serve your plate of food at the stove or kitchen counter. Do not put the serving dishes on the table. If you do put dishes on the table, remove them immediately when finished eating. Fill half of your plate with vegetables, a quarter with lean protein and a quarter with starch.

> Use smaller plates, bowls, and glasses. A smaller portion will look large when it is in a little dish. Politely refuse second helpings. When fixing your plate, limit portions of food to one scoop/serving or less.

Daily Food Management:

> Replace eating with another activity that you will not associate with food. Wait 20 minutes before eating something you are craving. Drink a large glass of water or diet soda before eating.

> Always have a big glass or bottle of water to drink throughout the day. Avoid high-calorie add-ons such as cream with your coffee, butter, mayonnaise, and salad dressings.

Shopping:

> Do not shop when hungry or tired. Shop from a list and avoid buying anything that is not on your list. If you must have tempting foods, buy individual-sized packages and try to find a lower-calorie alternative.

> Do not taste test in the store. Read food labels. Compare products to help you make the healthiest choices.

Preparation:

> Chew a piece of gum while cooking meals. Use a quarter teaspoon if you taste test your food. Try to only fix what you are going to eat, leaving yourself no chance for seconds.

> If you have prepared more food than you need, portion it into individual containers and freeze or refrigerate immediately. Do not snack while cooking meals.

Eating:

❯ Eat slowly. Remember it takes about 20 minutes for your stomach to send a message to your brain that it is full. Do not let fake hunger make you think you need more. The ideal way to eat is to take a bite, put your utensil down, take a sip of water, cut your next bite, take a bit, put your utensil down and so on.

❯ Do not cut your food all at one time. Cut only as needed. Take small bites and chew your food well. Stop eating for a minute or two at least once during a meal or snack. Take breaks to reflect and have conversation.

Cleanup and Leftovers:

❯ Label leftovers for a specific meal or snack. Freeze or refrigerate individual portions of leftovers.

❯ Do not clean up if you are still hungry.

Eating Out and Social Eating:

❯ Do not arrive hungry. Eat something light before the meal. Try to fill up on low-calorie foods, such as vegetables and fruit, and eat smaller portions of the high-calorie foods.

❯ Eat foods that you like but choose small portions.

❯ If you want seconds, wait at least 20 minutes after you have eaten to see if you are still hungry. Limit alcoholic beverages. Try a soda water with a twist of lime. Do not skip other meals in the day to save room for the special event.

At Restaurants:

❯ Order à la carte rather than buffet style. Order some vegetables or a salad for an appetizer instead of eating bread. If you order a high-calorie dish, share it with someone.

❯ Try an after-dinner mint with your coffee. If you do have dessert, share it with two or more people.

❯ Do not overeat because you do not want to waste food. Ask for a doggie bag to take extra food home.

❯ Tell the server to put half of your entree in a to go bag before the meal is served to you.

❯ Ask for salad dressing, gravy, or high-fat sauces on the side. Dip the tip of your fork in the dressing before each bite.

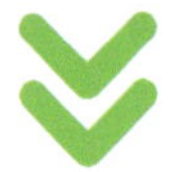

> If bread is served, ask for only one piece. Try it plain without butter or oil. At Italian restaurants where oil and vinegar are served with bread, use only a small amount of oil and a lot of vinegar for dipping.

At a Friend's House:

> Offer to bring a dish, appetizer or dessert that is low in calories. Serve yourself small portions or tell the host that you only want a small amount.

> Stand or sit away from the snack table. Stay away from the kitchen or stay busy if you are near the food.

> Limit your alcohol intake.

At Buffets and Cafeterias:

> Cover most of your plate with lettuce and/or vegetables. Use a salad plate instead of a dinner plate.

> After eating, clear away your dishes before having coffee or tea.

Entertaining at Home:

> Explore low-fat, low-cholesterol cookbooks. Use single-serving foods like chicken breasts or hamburger patties.

> Prepare low-calorie appetizers and desserts.

Holidays:

> Keep tempting foods out of sight. Decorate the house without using food. Have low-calorie beverages and foods on hand for guests.

> Allow yourself one planned treat a day.

> Do not skip meals to save up for the holiday feast.

> Eat regular, planned meals.

Exercise Well:

> Make exercise a priority and a planned activity in the day. If possible, walk the entire or part of the distance to work. Get an exercise buddy. Go for a walk with a colleague during one of your breaks, go to the gym, run, or take a walk with a friend, walk in the mall with a shopping companion.

> Park at the end of the parking lot and walk to the store or office entrance. Always take the stairs all the way or at least part of the way to

your floor. If you have a desk job, walk around the office frequently. Do leg lifts while sitting at your desk. Do something outside on the week-ends like going for a hike or a bike ride.

Have a Healthy Attitude:

> Make health your weight management priority. Be realistic. Have a goal to achieve a healthier you, not necessarily the lowest weight or ideal weight based on calculations or tables.

> Focus on a healthy eating style, not on dieting. Dieting usually lasts for a short amount of time and rarely produces long-term success.

> Think long term. You are developing new healthy behaviors to follow next month, in a year and in a decade.

*Transforming your habits is the first
step to transforming your life.
Small, consistent changes
lead to monumental results.*

The Effects of Stress on the Body

Stress is a natural response to challenging situations, but when it becomes chronic, it can have a profound impact on both your physical and mental health. When you're stressed, your body releases hormones like cortisol and adrenaline, which prepare you for a "fight or flight" response.

While this can be beneficial in short bursts, prolonged stress can lead to a host of health problems, including headaches, muscle tension, digestive issues, sleep disturbances, and a weakened immune system. Over time, chronic stress can also contribute to the development of more serious conditions such as heart disease, high blood pressure, and diabetes.

How Stress Affects Weight Loss

Stress can be a significant barrier to weight loss. Elevated cortisol levels, which are a hallmark of chronic stress, can lead to increased appetite and cravings for high-calorie, sugary, and fatty foods. This is often referred to as "stress eating," where individuals seek comfort in food as a way to cope with their emotions. Additionally, cortisol can lead to the accumulation of abdominal fat, which is particularly harmful to health. Stress also disrupts sleep patterns, and poor sleep is closely linked to weight gain. Furthermore, stress can sap your motivation to exercise and make it harder to stick to a healthy eating plan.

Signs of Experiencing Stress

Recognizing the signs of stress is the first step in managing it effectively. Common signs include:

> Physical Symptoms: Headaches, muscle tension, fatigue, chest pain, digestive problems.

> Emotional Symptoms: Anxiety, irritability, depression, feeling overwhelmed.

> Cognitive Symptoms: Difficulty concentrating, forgetfulness, negative thoughts.

> Behavioral Symptoms: Changes in appetite, sleep disturbances, with-drawing from social interactions, increased use of alcohol or drugs.

Practical Tips and Strategies to Handle Stress

Managing stress is crucial for overall well-being and can significantly aid in weight loss efforts. Here are some practical strategies to help you handle stress:

a. Exercise Regularly: Physical activity is one of the most effective ways to reduce stress. Exercise releases endorphins, which are natural mood lifters, and helps lower cortisol levels. Even a brisk walk or a yoga session can make a big difference.

b. Practice Mindfulness and Meditation: Mindfulness techniques, such as meditation, deep breathing, and progressive muscle relaxation, can help calm the mind and reduce stress. Spending just a few minutes each day on these practices can improve your resilience to stress.

c. Prioritize Sleep: Adequate sleep is essential for stress management. Aim for 7-9 hours of quality sleep each night. Establish a regular sleep routine, avoid screens before bedtime, and create a relaxing sleep environment.

d. Healthy Diet: Eating a balanced diet can help stabilize your mood and energy levels. Include plenty of fruits, vegetables, lean proteins, and whole grains. Avoid excessive caffeine, sugar, and alcohol, as these can exacerbate stress.

e. Stay Connected: Social support is vital in managing stress. Talk to friends, family, or a counselor about your stressors. Sometimes, just sharing your feelings can make them seem more manageable.

f. Time Management: Organize your tasks and prioritize what's most important. Break large tasks into smaller, manageable steps, and don't be afraid to delegate when possible.

g. Hobbies and Relaxation: Engage in activities that you enjoy and that help you relax. Whether it's reading, gardening, or listening to music, finding time for relaxation can reduce stress.

h. Deep Breathing: Breathe from your stomach. Draw in a deep breath through your nose. Feel your lungs expand, hold your breath for three seconds and then let the breath out slowly through your mouth. Keep doing this for three to five minutes.

i. Letting your mind wander: Set aside 15 minutes a day to clear your mind and let your thoughts wander. Do this in a quiet place. Close your eyes and try not to think of anything.

j. Limit Exposure to Stress Triggers: If possible, identify and minimize exposure to stressors in your life, whether it's work-related or personal. Setting boundaries and learning to say no can be powerful tools.

Supplements That Can Be Beneficial

Certain supplements can support the body during periods of stress and promote overall well-being:

a. Ashwagandha: An adaptogenic herb known for its ability to reduce stress and anxiety by lowering cortisol levels.

b. Magnesium: This mineral is essential for relaxation and helps regulate the nervous system. It's known to alleviate symptoms of stress and improve sleep quality.

c. B-Complex Vitamins: B vitamins, particularly B6 and B12, are important for energy production and nervous system health. They can help reduce stress and improve mood.

d. L-Theanine: An amino acid found in green tea, L-theanine promotes relaxation without causing drowsiness. It's known to enhance focus and reduce the physical symptoms of stress.

e. Omega-3 Fatty Acids: Found in fish oil, omega-3s have anti-inflammatory properties and can help reduce stress-related inflammation and improve mood.

f. Rhodiola Rosea: Another adaptogen, Rhodiola, is known for its ability to enhance the body's resistance to stress and improve mental performance and stamina.

g. Valerian Root: Often used as a natural remedy for anxiety and sleep disorders, Valerian can help with relaxation and stress relief.

h. Probiotics: A healthy gut can influence stress levels, as the gut-brain axis plays a role in mood regulation. Probiotic supplements can support gut health, which in turn can help manage stress.

By addressing stress through these practical strategies and incorporating supportive supplements, you can create a balanced approach to weight loss that not only helps you achieve your goals but also enhances your overall quality of life.

What does sleep have to do with weight loss?

Sleep is a crucial factor in your weight loss journey! Getting enough quality sleep is a vital component of a successful weight loss strategy and overall health.

By regulating hunger hormones, reducing cravings, boosting metabolism, supporting physical activity, and improving decision-making, sleep plays a fundamental role in helping you achieve and maintain a healthy weight. Prioritizing sleep alongside a balanced diet and regular exercise will enhance your overall health and well-being, making your weight loss journey more effective and sustainable.

Here's how getting adequate, quality sleep can support your weight loss efforts:

> **Regulates Hunger Hormones:** Sleep helps balance the hormones that control hunger—ghrelin and leptin. Ghrelin stimulates appetite, while leptin signals fullness. Lack of sleep increases ghrelin levels and decreases leptin levels, leading to increased hunger and appetite, especially for high-calorie foods.

> **Reduces Cravings and Late-Night Snacking:** Poor sleep can increase cravings for sugary, fatty, and carbohydrate-rich foods. This is partly due to hormonal imbalances and the body's attempt to find quick energy sources. Adequate sleep helps regulate these cravings, reducing the likelihood of overeating or indulging in late-night snacks.

> **Boosts Metabolism:** Sleep deprivation can negatively impact your metabolism. It can lead to insulin resistance, making it harder for your body to process glucose, which can contribute to weight gain. Quality sleep helps maintain a healthy metabolism and improves insulin sensitivity.

> **Supports Physical Activity:** Being well-rested improves your energy levels and physical performance, making it easier to stick to your exercise routine. When you're tired, you're less likely to exercise, and your workouts may be less effective.

> **Enhances Recovery:** Sleep is essential for muscle recovery and growth. During deep sleep, your body repairs and builds muscle tissue.

More muscle mass boosts your resting metabolic rate, helping you burn more calories even at rest.

> **Reduces Stress:** Sleep helps regulate the stress hormone cortisol. Chronic sleep deprivation can lead to elevated cortisol levels, which are associated with increased appetite and fat storage, particularly in the abdominal area. Lower cortisol levels due to adequate sleep can aid in reducing stress-related eating and weight gain.

> **Improves Decision-Making:** Lack of sleep impairs cognitive function and decision-making, making it harder to choose healthy foods and stick to your diet plan. Being well-rested helps you make better food choices and resist unhealthy temptations.

> **Supports Emotional Health:** Poor sleep can affect your mood and lead to emotional eating. Adequate sleep helps regulate your emotions, reducing the likelihood of turning to food for comfort.

> **Regulates Blood Sugar Levels:** Consistent, quality sleep helps stabilize blood sugar levels. Fluctuating blood sugar can lead to increased hunger and cravings, making it harder to control your diet.

> **Maintains Overall Health:** Good sleep supports overall health, including immune function, heart health, and brain function. A healthy body is better equipped to manage weight effectively.

Tips for Better Sleep

> **Establish a Routine:** Go to bed and wake up at the same time every day, even on weekends, to regulate your internal clock.

> **Create a Sleep-Friendly Environment:** Keep your bedroom cool, dark, and quiet. Invest in a comfortable mattress and pillows.

> **Limit Screen Time:** Avoid screens (phones, tablets, computers, TV) at least an hour before bed, as the blue light can disrupt your sleep cycle.

> **Watch Your Diet:** Avoid heavy meals, caffeine, and alcohol close to bedtime. These can interfere with your ability to fall and stay asleep.

> **Exercise Regularly:** Physical activity can help you fall asleep faster and enjoy deeper sleep. Just avoid vigorous exercise close to bedtime.

> **Manage Stress:** Incorporate relaxation techniques such as deep breathing, meditation, or gentle yoga before bed to reduce stress.

> **Limit Naps:** If you need to nap, keep it short (20-30 minutes) and avoid napping late in the afternoon.

> **Stay Hydrated:** Drink enough water throughout the day but reduce fluid intake in the evening to minimize nighttime trips to the bathroom.

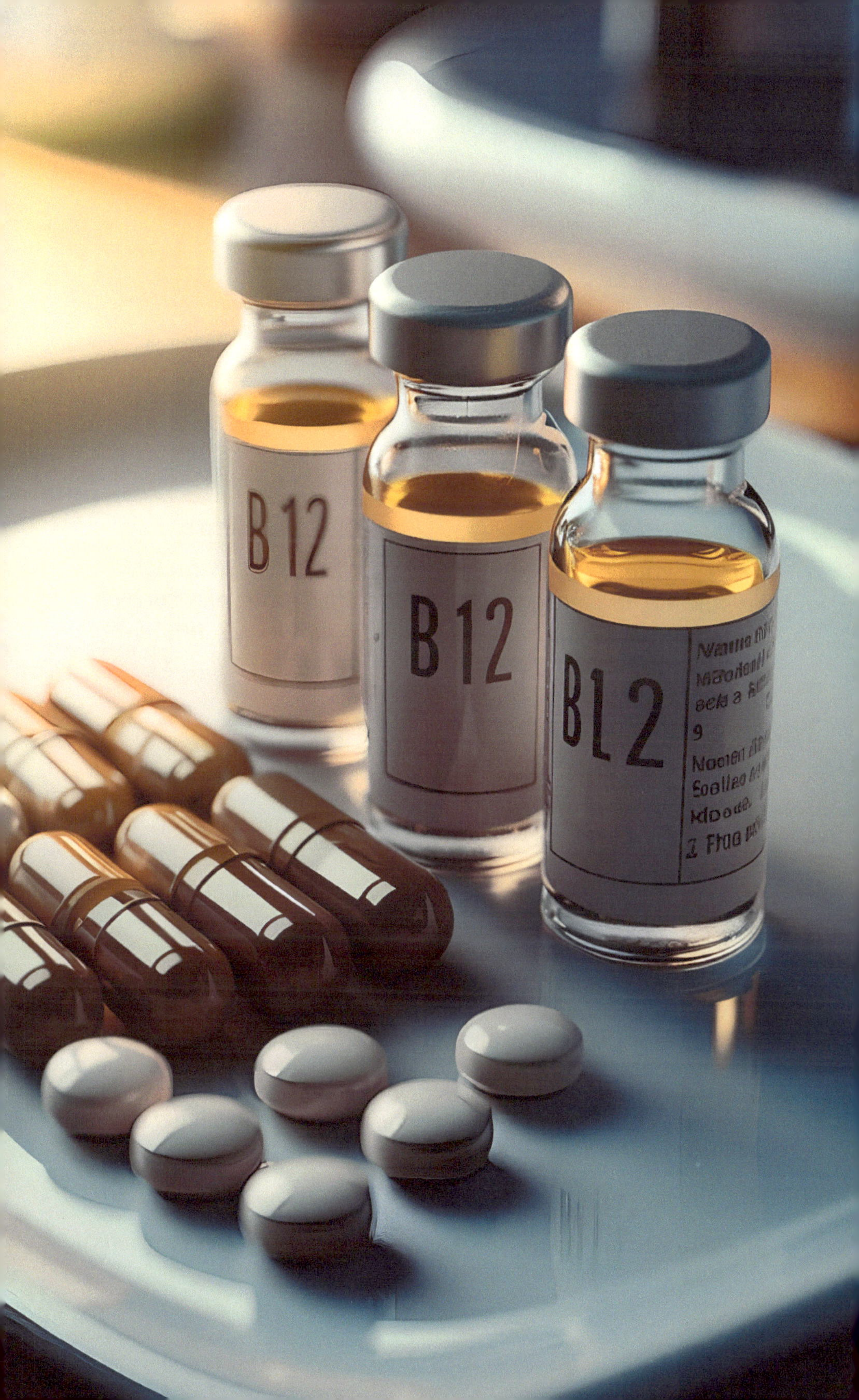

B 12
B 12
B 12

The Importance of Supplementation with Lipotropics and Other Nutrients for Weight Loss

In the quest for effective weight loss, supplementation can play a crucial role in supporting metabolic functions, enhancing fat burning, and ensuring overall health. Lipotropics such as Lipolean, MIC (Methionine, Inositol, Choline), B12, Chromium Picolinate, Calcium Pyruvate, multivitamins, and detox supplements are among the most beneficial.

Here's a closer look at their importance and how they can aid in your weight loss journey:

1. Lipolean

Lipolean is a combination of lipotropic agents designed to promote fat loss by enhancing liver function and increasing the body's ability to metabolize fat. It typically contains ingredients like methionine, inositol, and choline, which support the breakdown and elimination of fat. It also contains B vitamins, amino acids and L-Carnite that are necessary for the maintenance of a healthy liver as well as burning the exported fat for additional energy. This injection helps you to lose weight by boosting energy so that you will burn off more calories, increasing the removal of fat from the body, and overall health and wellness on our program.

2. MIC (Methionine, Inositol, Choline)

The MIC injection is a popular supplement in weight loss programs due to its powerful lipotropic effects.

> Methionine: Supports the detoxification process and aids in the elimination of heavy metals, boosting liver health and fat metabolism.

> Inositol: Improves the body's use of insulin, enhancing fat burning and energy levels.

> Choline: Essential for liver function and fat utilization, preventing fat buildup in the liver.

3. Vitamin B12

Vitamin B12 is a water-soluble vitamin that plays a vital role in energy production and metabolism.

> **Energy Boost:** B12 helps convert food into glucose, providing energy and reducing fatigue, which is crucial for maintaining an active lifestyle.

> **Metabolism Support:** It aids in the metabolism of fats and proteins, supporting weight loss efforts.

> **Mood Regulation:** B12 supports the nervous system and can improve mood and cognitive function, reducing stress-related eating.

4. Chromium Picolinate

Chromium Picolinate is a mineral that enhances insulin sensitivity and helps regulate blood sugar levels.

> **Blood Sugar Control:** Improves insulin function, reducing cravings for sugary and carbohydrate-rich foods.

> **Appetite Regulation:** Can help reduce hunger and control appetite, making it easier to stick to a calorie-controlled diet.

> **Fat Loss:** Supports the metabolism of fats and carbohydrates, aiding in weight loss.

5. Calcium Pyruvate

Calcium Pyruvate is a naturally occurring substance that plays a key role in the body's energy production.

> **Increased Metabolism:** Enhances the body's ability to burn fat by improving the efficiency of the Krebs cycle, the process by which cells produce energy.

> **Improved Exercise Performance:** Provides more energy, helping to enhance physical performance and endurance during workouts.

> **Fat Reduction:** Can aid in reducing body fat while preserving lean muscle mass.

6. Multivitamins

A comprehensive multivitamin ensures that the body receives all essential vitamins and minerals required for optimal health.

> **Nutrient Deficiency Prevention:** Ensures that the body gets a balanced intake of nutrients, which can be challenging with a restricted diet.

> **Immune Support:** Boosts the immune system, helping to maintain health and prevent illness.

> **Energy Levels:** Provides the necessary vitamins and minerals to support overall energy and well-being.

7. Detox Supplements

Detox supplements help support the body's natural detoxification processes, promoting the elimination of toxins and improving metabolic health.

> **Liver Health:** Ingredients like milk thistle and dandelion root support liver function, aiding in the detoxification of the body.

> **Digestive Health:** Helps improve digestion and nutrient absorption, which is crucial for maintaining energy levels and overall health.

> **Weight Loss Support:** By reducing the toxic load in the body, detox supplements can enhance the efficiency of metabolic processes and support weight loss.

Integrating Supplements into Your Weight Loss Plan

To maximize the benefits of these supplements, it's important to integrate them into a comprehensive weight loss plan that includes a balanced diet, regular exercise, and lifestyle modifications. Here's how to do it effectively:

1. **Consult a Healthcare Professional:** Before starting any supplementation regimen, consult with one of our healthcare providers to ensure it's appropriate for your individual health needs and goals.

2. **Follow Recommended Dosages:** Adhere to the recommended dosages and guidelines provided by our healthcare provider or the product manufacturer.

3. Maintain a Balanced Diet: Supplements should complement, not replace, a healthy diet rich in whole foods, lean proteins, healthy fats, and a variety of fruits and vegetables.

4. Stay Hydrated: Drink plenty of water to support the body's detoxification processes and overall metabolic function.

5. Exercise Regularly: Combine supplementation with a consistent exercise routine that includes both cardiovascular and strength-training activities.

6. Monitor Progress: Keep track of your weight loss progress and any changes in how you feel. Adjust your supplementation and lifestyle habits as needed.

Supplementation with lipotropics and other supportive nutrients can play a significant role in enhancing weight loss efforts. By boosting metabolism, supporting fat breakdown, regulating appetite, and ensuring overall nutritional balance, these supplements can help overcome plateaus and accelerate progress. However, they should be used as part of a holistic approach to weight loss that includes a healthy diet, regular exercise, and lifestyle modifications. Always consult with one of our knowledgeable healthcare providers before starting any new supplement regimen to ensure it aligns with your health needs and goals.

Semaglutide and Tirzepatide: The Game Changers

In the quest for effective weight loss, supplementation can play a crucial role in supporting metabolic functions, enhancing fat burning, and ensuring overall health. Lipotropics such as Lipolean, MIC (Methionine, Inositol, Choline), B12, Chromium Picolinate, Calcium Pyruvate, multivitamins, and detox supplements are among the most beneficial.

Semaglutide and Tirzepatide are groundbreaking medications that have gained significant attention for their effectiveness in managing weight loss, especially in individuals who struggle with obesity or have difficulty losing weight through diet and exercise alone. Both medications belong to a class of drugs known as GLP-1 (glucagon-like peptide-1) receptor agonists, though Tirzepatide has dual activity, also acting as a GIP (glucose-dependent insulinotropic polypeptide) receptor agonist. Semaglutide has been approved for weight loss by the FDA under the brand name Wegovy (Ozempic for type 2 diabetes) while Tirzepatide was recently approved for weight loss under the brand name Zepbound (Mounjaro for type 2 diabetes).

Before starting Semaglutide or Tirzepatide, it is crucial to undergo a thorough medical evaluation by a healthcare provider to determine if these medications are appropriate for you. They are generally safe and effective when used under medical supervision, but due to the potential risks and contraindications, they should only be taken with a prescription and close monitoring by a healthcare professional.

How Semaglutide Works

Semaglutide mimics the action of the naturally occurring hormone GLP-1, which is involved in regulating appetite and food intake. By activating GLP-1 receptors in the brain, Semaglutide helps to:

❯ **Reduce Appetite:** It slows down the movement of food through the stomach, making you feel full for longer periods, which naturally reduces the amount of food you consume.

❯ **Control Cravings:** By influencing the brain's appetite control center, Semaglutide helps reduce cravings and the desire to snack between meals.

❯ **Improve Blood Sugar Levels:** Semaglutide enhances insulin secretion in response to high blood sugar levels, helping to maintain better glucose control, which is often a challenge for people with obesity or type 2 diabetes.

The combination of these effects leads to a significant reduction in overall calorie intake, which can result in substantial weight loss over time.

How Tirzepatide Works

Tirzepatide is a dual agonist that targets both GLP-1 and GIP receptors, offering a more comprehensive approach to weight loss and metabolic regulation. It works through the following mechanisms: It is worthy to note that significant weight loss has been noted to occur in patients who inject Tirzepatide when compared with outcomes of weight lost with those who used Semaglutide.

❯ **Dual Hormonal Action:** By activating both GLP-1 and GIP receptors, Tirzepatide enhances insulin secretion, improves insulin sensitivity, and reduces glucagon levels, which helps regulate blood sugar more effectively than GLP-1 agonists alone.

❯ **Enhanced Appetite Suppression:** Like Semaglutide, Tirzepatide slows gastric emptying and affects the brain's hunger signals, leading to a decrease in appetite and calorie intake.

❯ **Increased Fat Loss:** Tirzepatide has been shown to specifically target fat mass, helping to reduce body fat while preserving lean muscle mass, which is crucial for long-term weight management.

How These Medications Help with Weight Loss

Both Semaglutide and Tirzepatide have been proven in clinical trials to result in significant weight loss, often exceeding the results of traditional diet and exercise programs alone or even Phentermine alone or Phentermine plus Topiramate. Here's how they contribute to effective weight management:

❯ **Sustained Satiety:** By slowing the emptying of the stomach, both drugs help you feel fuller longer, reducing the frequency and intensity of hunger pangs.

> **Reduced Caloric Intake:** The decrease in appetite and control of cravings lead to a natural reduction in calorie consumption, which is essential for weight loss.

> **Improved Metabolism:** These medications improve metabolic efficiency, allowing the body to process nutrients more effectively and burn fat more readily.

> **Better Blood Sugar Control:** For individuals with type 2 diabetes or insulin resistance, these medications help regulate blood sugar levels, which can indirectly support weight loss by reducing insulin-related fat storage.

Who Can Benefit

Semaglutide and Tirzepatide are typically prescribed for individuals with a body mass index (BMI) of 30 or higher with no weight-related complications (or 27 or higher with related health conditions such as type 2 diabetes, high blood pressure or high cholesterol). They are particularly beneficial for those who have struggled to lose weight through conventional methods alone.

Contraindications:

There are several contraindications and precautions to consider when using Semaglutide or Tirzepatide for weight loss. These medications, while effective, are not suitable for everyone. Here are the major key contraindications:

Personal or Family History of Medullary Thyroid Carcinoma (MTC)

> Semaglutide and Tirzepatide are contraindicated in individuals with a personal or family history of medullary thyroid carcinoma, a type of thyroid cancer. This is due to the potential risk of developing thyroid tumors.

Multiple Endocrine Neoplasia Syndrome Type 2 (MEN 2)

> These medications are also contraindicated in individuals with Multiple Endocrine Neoplasia syndrome type 2, a genetic condition that increases the risk of developing tumors in endocrine glands.

Precautions:

> Severe Gastrointestinal Disease

People with severe gastrointestinal diseases, such as gastroparesis (delayed stomach emptying), should avoid these medications. Both Semaglutide and Tirzepatide slow gastric emptying, which could exacerbate these conditions.

Pancreatitis

There have been reports of pancreatitis (inflammation of the pancreas) in people using GLP-1 receptor agonists. Individuals with a history of pancreatitis should use these medications with caution or avoid them altogether.

Hypersensitivity Reactions

Individuals who have had an allergic or hypersensitivity reaction to Semaglutide, Tirzepatide, or any of the excipients in the formulations should not use these medications. You must discontinue using any GLP-1and get medical help right away, if you have any symptoms of a serious allergic reaction, including swelling of your face, lips, tongue, or throat; problems breathing or swallowing; severe rash or itching; fainting or feeling dizzy; or very rapid heartbeat.

Pregnancy and Breastfeeding

These medications are not recommended for use during pregnancy due to the potential risk to the fetus. They should also be avoided during breastfeeding, as it is unknown if they pass into breast milk.

Severe Kidney or Liver Disease

Caution is advised in individuals with severe kidney or liver disease. While Semaglutide and Tirzepatide can be used in patients with mild to moderate kidney or liver impairment, those with severe conditions should be closely monitored or avoid these medications. In people who have kidney problems, diarrhea, nausea, and vomiting may cause a loss of fluids (dehydration) which may cause kidney problems to get worse. It is important for you to drink fluids to help reduce your chance of dehydration. Adequate hydration is required during your treatment.

Hypoglycemia Risk in Combination with Insulin or Sulfonylureas

While Semaglutide and Tirzepatide themselves are not typically associated with hypoglycemia, the risk increases when used in combination with insulin or sulfonylureas (a type of oral diabetes medication). Dosage adjustments of these other medications may be necessary to avoid low blood sugar. This can be both a serious and common side effect. Talk to your healthcare provider about how to recognize and treat low blood sugar and check your blood sugar before you start taking any GLP-1. Signs and symptoms of low blood sugar may include dizziness or light-headedness, blurred vision, anxiety, irritability, or mood changes, sweating, slurred speech, hunger, confusion or drowsiness, shakiness, weakness, headache, fast heartbeat, or feeling jittery.

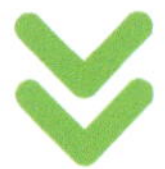

> Personal or Family History of Diabetic Retinopathy

Semaglutide has been associated with worsening diabetic retinopathy in some individuals. Those with a history of this eye condition should use the medication cautiously and under close supervision by their healthcare provider.

> Drug Interactions

Both medications can interact with other drugs, potentially altering their effectiveness or increasing the risk of side effects. For example, they may affect the absorption of oral medications that require rapid gastric emptying. It's important to discuss all current medications with a healthcare provider before starting Semaglutide or Tirzepatide.

> Increased heart rate

GLP-1s can increase your heart rate while you are at rest. Inform your healthcare provider if you feel your heart racing or pounding in your chest and it lasts for several minutes.

> Depression or thoughts of suicide

You should pay attention to any mental changes, especially sudden changes in your mood, behaviors, thoughts, or feelings. Call your healthcare provider right away if you have any mental changes that are new, worse, or bothersome.

GLP-1/ GIP Injection Instructions:

1. You will only take the shot once a week. Pick a day that you will re-member to take it, not to get off schedule. Inject 30 minutes before or after any other medications or vitamins. It does not matter what time of day you take it. Just be consistent!

2. Your dose each week may vary.

3. Each week, one time per week, you will inject the prescribed amount.

4. Pinch fat in your belly/abdominal area or other parts as shown be-low, clean with alcohol and give yourself an injection.

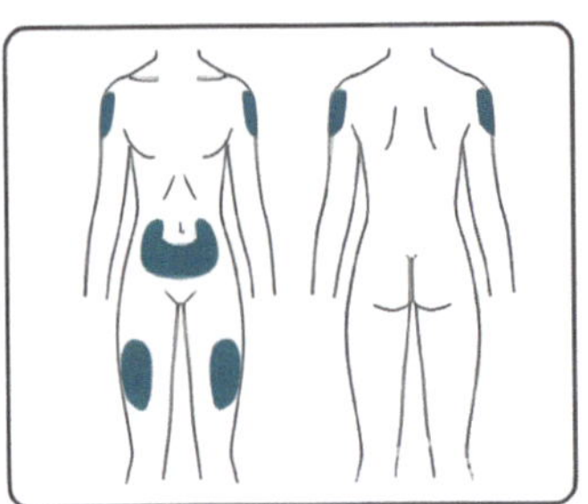

> Do not use the same site for each injection.

> If you choose to inject in the same area, always use a different spot in that area.

5. Refrigerate your medication and keep it in a safe and dry place.

6. Store your medication in a refrigerator between 36°F to 46°F (2°C to 8°C).

7. Keep away from heat and out of the light.

8. If you have a vial, it will break if it is dropped.

9. If you miss a dose, take the missed dose as soon as possible within 4 days after the missed dose.

10. Keep GLP-1 and all medicines out of the reach of children.

11. Your dose will most likely increase after the 1st month.

12. If you do not tolerate the dose, please inform your healthcare provider for adjustments.

13. Do not reuse your needles. Use a clean syringe each time or just inject as dispensed. Dispose of your needles properly by using a hard plastic container such as a milk jug or 2-liter bottle to place your needles in for disposal.

Common Side Effects of Semaglutide and Tirzepatide and How to Manage Them

Both Semaglutide and Tirzepatide are effective for weight loss and blood sugar control, but like all medications, they come with potential side effects. Here are some of the most common side effects and strategies for managing them:

Nausea

Nausea is one of the most frequently reported side effects, especially when starting the medication or increasing the dose.

Management:

> **Gradual Dose Increase:** Start with the lowest dose and gradually increase it as recommended by your healthcare provider to help your body adjust.

> **Eat Smaller, More Frequent Meals:** Avoid large meals, which can exacerbate nausea. Opt for smaller, more frequent meals instead.

> **Avoid Rich, fried or Fatty Foods:** These can make nausea worse. Stick to lighter, bland foods if nausea occurs.

> **Hydrate:** Drinking water in small sips throughout the day can help alleviate nausea.

> Eat foods that contain water like low-salt soups and sugar-free gelatin.

> Avoid lying down after you eat.

> Go outdoors for fresh air.

> Eat low fat meal or bland diet-bananas, rice, toast

> Consider injecting your medication just before bedtime

> You can inject the GLP-1 in your thigh or arm to slow down absorption and nausea

> Take Ginger or Vitamin B6 for nausea

> Your healthcare provider can prescribe anti-nausea medication such as Zofran

Diarrhea

Diarrhea is another common gastrointestinal side effect.

Management:

> Stay Hydrated: Drink plenty of fluids to avoid dehydration. Oral rehydration solutions or clear broths can be helpful.

> Avoid Trigger Foods: Fatty, fried, or spicy foods can worsen diarrhea. Stick to a bland diet if diarrhea occurs.

> Consider Probiotics: These may help restore the balance of good bacteria in your gut. Consult with your healthcare provider before starting probiotics.

Vomiting

Vomiting can occur, particularly if the dose is increased too quickly.

Management:

> Slow Dose Titration: Increase the dose slowly as advised by your healthcare provider to minimize this risk.

> Eat Light: Stick to light, easy-to-digest foods and avoid overeating.

> Anti-Nausea Medications: Over-the-counter or prescription anti-nausea medications can be used if vomiting is persistent. Consult your healthcare provider before using them.

Constipation

Constipation can occur, although it is less common than other gastrointestinal side effects.

Management:

> Increase Fiber Intake: Include more high-fiber foods like vegetables, fruits, and whole grains in your diet.

> Stay Hydrated: Drink plenty of water to help keep your digestive system moving.

> Regular Exercise: Physical activity can help stimulate digestion and prevent constipation.

> Take daily stool softeners like Miralax, Colace or Senna laxative.

Abdominal Pain

Some people may experience abdominal discomfort or pain.

Management:

> Avoid Heavy Meals: Eating smaller, more frequent meals can help reduce abdominal discomfort.

> Use a Heating Pad: Applying heat to the abdomen can help alleviate discomfort.

> Consult Your Healthcare Provider: If the pain is severe or persistent, it's important to consult your healthcare provider and seek medical care, as this may indicate a more serious issue.

Headache

Headaches can occur, particularly when starting the medication.

Management:

> Stay Hydrated: Dehydration can contribute to headaches, so be sure to drink plenty of water.

> Rest: Ensure you get adequate sleep and take breaks if you're feeling overwhelmed.

> Over-the-Counter Pain Relief: Mild headaches can often be managed with over-the-counter pain relievers like Acetaminophen or Ibuprofen, but consult your healthcare provider first.

Fatigue

Some individuals may feel more tired than usual when starting the medication.

Management:

> Balanced Diet: Ensure you're getting adequate nutrition, as low energy can sometimes result from poor diet.

> Regular Exercise: Light physical activity can boost your energy levels.

> Adequate Rest: Ensure you're getting enough sleep to help manage fatigue.

> Vitamin B12 shots can be helpful to boost your energy levels.

Injection Site Reactions (if injected)

Mild redness, swelling, or irritation can occur at the injection site.

Management:

❯ Rotate Injection Sites: Avoid using the same injection site repeatedly. Rotate between different areas to minimize irritation.

❯ Use Proper Technique: Ensure you are using the correct injection technique as instructed by your healthcare provider.

❯ Apply a Cool Compress: If you experience redness or swelling, applying a cool compress to the area can help reduce inflammation.

Hypoglycemia (Low Blood Sugar)

Although less common, hypoglycemia can occur, especially if you are taking other diabetes medications like insulin or sulfonylureas.

Management:

❯ Monitor Blood Sugar: Regularly check your blood sugar levels to ensure they are within the target range.

❯ Carry Quick-Acting Carbohydrates: Keep glucose tablets, candy, or juice with you in case of low blood sugar episodes.

❯ Adjust Other Medications: Consult your healthcare provider about adjusting the dosage of other diabetes medications to reduce the risk of hypoglycemia.

While Semaglutide and Tirzepatide are generally well-tolerated, side effects can occur. Most side effects are mild and can be managed with lifestyle adjustments and by following your healthcare provider's guidance. If side effects persist or worsen, it's important to contact your healthcare provider, as they may need to adjust your dosage or explore other treatment options.

The Power of GLP-1 and the Ultimate Guide

Combining Semaglutide or Tirzepatide with "The Ultimate Guide to Lasting Weight Loss" offers a powerful and comprehensive approach to achieving sustainable weight loss. Here's how you can benefit from this combination:

Enhanced Weight Loss Results

❯ Medication's Role: Semaglutide and Tirzepatide are proven to significantly reduce appetite, control cravings, and improve metabolism, leading to more effective and sustained weight loss.

❯ Guide's Role: "The Ultimate Guide to Lasting Weight Loss" provides the dietary guidelines, exercise routines, and behavior modification strategies that maximize the effects of these medications. The structured approach in the guide helps you make the most out of your medication, leading to faster and more substantial results.

Comprehensive Support

❯ Medication's Role: These medications work on a physiological level, addressing hunger hormones and insulin sensitivity to make weight loss more manageable.

❯ Guide's Role: The guide offers practical tips, sample menus, and strategies for overcoming challenges like plateaus, making it easier to stay on track with your weight loss journey. It also provides behavioral tools to change your mindset and habits, ensuring that the weight you lose is lost for good.

Personalized Approach

❯ Medication's Role: Both Semaglutide and Tirzepatide can be tailored to your specific health needs, ensuring you receive the optimal dosage for your weight loss goals.

❯ Guide's Role: The book allows you to personalize your weight loss journey by choosing the foods, exercises, and strategies that work best for you. When combined with medication, this tailored approach enhances your ability to achieve and maintain your ideal weight.

Long-Term Success

❯ Medication's Role: These medications not only help you lose weight but also improve overall metabolic health, reducing the risk of weight regain.

❯ Guide's Role: "The Ultimate Guide to Lasting Weight Loss" emphasizes the importance of maintenance strategies, including a gradual weaning off the medication and the adoption of healthy habits that support long-term success. The guide ensures that once you've reached your goal weight, you're equipped with the knowledge and skills to maintain it.

Holistic Well-Being

❯ Medication's Role: By controlling blood sugar levels and reducing fat mass, these medications contribute to overall health improvements, including better cardiovascular health and reduced risk of diabetes.

❯ Guide's Role: The guide addresses all aspects of well-being, including mental health, stress management, and behavior modification, creating a holistic approach to weight loss that goes beyond just the physical. This combination promotes not just a healthier body but a healthier mind as well.

Overcoming Plateaus

❯ Medication's Role: Semaglutide and Tirzepatide can help you break through weight loss plateaus by continuing to suppress appetite and enhance metabolism even when progress slows.

❯ Guide's Role: The guide offers specific strategies for overcoming plateaus, such as adjusting your diet, intensifying your exercise routine, and employing mental strategies to stay motivated. When paired with medication, these strategies become even more effective.

Empowerment and Confidence

❯ Medication's Role: Seeing consistent weight loss results with the help of medication can boost your confidence and motivation to continue your journey.

> Guide's Role: The guide empowers you with the knowledge and tools to take control of your health. With Dr. Hilda's expertise and guidance, you'll feel more confident in your ability to achieve lasting weight loss.

Both Semaglutide and Tirzepatide represent a significant advancement in the medical management of obesity and weight-related health issues. By effectively reducing appetite, improving metabolic health, and promoting substantial weight loss, these medications offer new hope for individuals seeking lasting change. However, they should be used as part of a comprehensive weight loss plan that includes dietary changes, physical activity, and behavioral modifications, under the guidance of a healthcare professional.

By combining the physiological support of Semaglutide or Tirzepatide with the practical and motivational strategies in "The Ultimate Guide to Lasting Weight Loss," you create a powerful synergy that can lead to more significant and sustainable weight loss results. This combination not only helps you lose weight more effectively but also equips you with the skills and knowledge to maintain your success for the long term.

Why Do You Plateau on a Weight Loss Journey?

Weight loss plateaus are common and can be frustrating. It is a natural process because of the appetite signaling and hormonal changes that occur when you lose weight from any modality. Understanding why they happen and how to overcome them is crucial for continued progress.

The body goes through several processes to help us maintain our weight, which is why it might be frustrating to not be able to shed the last 5 pounds.

Here are some reasons why people plateau on their weight loss journey:

> **Metabolic Adaptation:** When you first start losing weight, your body burns calories more efficiently because it's adjusting to the new demands. However, over time, your body adapts to the lower calorie intake and exercise routine. This is called metabolic adaptation. And as you lose weight, your metabolism slows down to conserve energy, which can lead to a weight loss plateau—a point where your weight stays the same despite your efforts which can be frustrating. You may need to keep your body challenged to overcome a plateau by adjusting your diet, increasing your physical activity, or changing your exercise routine.

> **Loss of Muscle Mass:** Rapid weight loss can lead to the loss of muscle mass, which is metabolically active tissue. Less muscle mass means a slower metabolism.

> **Caloric Intake Mismatch:** Initially, a reduced-calorie diet leads to weight loss. Over time, however, the body adapts, and the same calorie intake may no longer result in a calorie deficit.

> **Inconsistent Diet and Exercise:** Gradual relaxation of dietary rules or exercise routines can lead to consuming more calories than intended or burning fewer calories.

> **Hormonal Changes:** Hormones like leptin, which regulates hunger and energy balance, can decrease with weight loss, leading to increased appetite and potential overeating.

> **Body's Set Point:** The body may resist weight loss by trying to maintain a certain weight, which it perceives as normal.

> **Inadequate Hydration:** Not drinking enough water can slow down metabolic processes and hinder weight loss.

> **Sleep Deprivation:** Lack of sleep can affect hunger hormones, leading to increased appetite and cravings.

> **Stress:** Chronic stress can lead to elevated cortisol levels, which may contribute to weight gain or hinder weight loss.

> **Lack of Variety in Exercise:** Performing the same exercise routine can lead to a plateau as your body becomes more efficient at these activities, burning fewer calories.

Strategies to Overcome a Weight Loss Plateau

> **Reassess Caloric Needs:** Recalculate your daily caloric needs based on your new weight. Adjust your calorie intake to create a new deficit.

> **Increase Protein Intake and Keto:** Protein can help preserve muscle mass during weight loss and boost metabolism. You can do a few days of the modified Ketogenic diet.

> **Change Your Exercise Routine:** Incorporate new types of exercises, increase the intensity, or add strength training to build muscle and boost metabolism.

> **Track Everything:** Keep a detailed food and exercise journal to identify any hidden calories or patterns that might be hindering progress.

> **Get Adequate Sleep:** Aim for 7-9 hours of quality sleep per night to support metabolic health and hormone balance.

> **Manage Stress:** Incorporate stress-reducing activities like meditation, yoga, or deep breathing exercises into your routine.

> **Stay Hydrated:** Drink plenty of water throughout the day to support metabolic functions and control hunger.

> **Consider Intermittent Fasting:** This eating pattern can help break through plateaus by changing when you eat, potentially leading to reduced calorie intake.

> **Reevaluate Macros:** Adjust the balance of carbohydrates, fats, and proteins in your diet. Sometimes tweaking your macronutrient ratio can help restart weight loss.

Implementing These Strategies

To effectively implement these strategies, it's important to approach them with patience and consistency. Here's a step-by-step plan:

> **Recalculate Your Needs:** Use an online calculator or consult a professional to determine your new caloric requirements.

> **Adjust Your Diet:** Increase your protein intake by incorporating lean meats, beans, and dairy. Reevaluate your portion sizes and cut back on high-calorie, low-nutrient foods.

> **Revamp Your Workouts:** Add strength training exercises to build muscle. Try high-intensity interval training (HIIT) to increase calorie burn.

> **Monitor and Record:** Use apps or journals to track your food intake and exercise. Identify any areas where you may be slipping.

> **Focus on Sleep and Stress:** Establish a regular sleep schedule and incorporate relaxation techniques into your daily routine.

> **Stay Hydrated and Healthy:** Drink at least 8 glasses of water a day. Avoid sugary drinks, alcohol and excessive caffeine.

> **Mix Up Your Routine:** Change your exercise routine every few weeks to keep your body challenged.

> **Stay Patient and Persistent:** Understand that plateaus are a normal part of the weight loss journey. Stay committed and keep pushing forward.

By understanding the reasons behind weight loss plateaus and implementing these strategies, you can overcome them and continue on your path to achieving your weight loss goals.

The Role of GLP-1 in Overcoming a Weight Loss Plateau

For you to get past that level of metabolic adaptability and break through a plateau, medications such as Semaglutide or Tirzepatide can be beneficial in overcoming a weight loss plateau. GLP-1, or glucagon-like peptide-1, assists with weight loss and particularly in overcoming weight loss plateaus. Here's how GLP-1 can help:

> **Appetite Suppression:** GLP-1 slows down gastric emptying and promotes a feeling of fullness, which can help reduce overall calorie intake. By curbing hunger, it helps individuals stick to their calorie goals more effectively, which is crucial when the body is resisting further weight loss.

> **Improved Blood Sugar Control:** GLP-1 helps to stabilize blood sugar levels by enhancing insulin secretion and inhibiting glucagon release after meals. Stable blood sugar levels can reduce cravings and the urge to snack between meals, which can be beneficial during a plateau.

> **Enhanced Satiety:** By enhancing feelings of satiety, GLP-1 can help individuals feel more satisfied with smaller portions, making it easier to adhere to a reduced-calorie diet.

> **Reduction in Food Intake:** GLP-1 receptors in the brain are involved in signaling satiety. Medications that mimic GLP-1, such as Tirzepatide and Semaglutide, can help reduce food intake, which is essential when trying to break through a weight loss plateau.

> **Promotion of Fat Loss:** GLP-1 can promote fat loss while preserving lean muscle mass. This is particularly important because muscle mass is metabolically active tissue that helps maintain a higher metabolic rate.

> **Regulation of Metabolism:** By improving insulin sensitivity and supporting better glucose utilization, GLP-1 can help optimize metabolism, making it easier to continue losing weight.

> **Behavioral Benefits:** GLP-1 medications can also help with behavior modification by reducing the reward response to food, which can help individuals make healthier food choices and resist high-calorie, low-nutrient foods.

> **Combination with Other Interventions:** GLP-1 therapy can be combined with dietary changes, increased physical activity, and behavior modification strategies to provide a comprehensive approach to overcoming weight loss plateaus.

Implementing GLP-1 Therapy

Overcoming a weight loss plateau requires a multifaceted approach, and GLP-1 therapy can be a valuable tool in this process. By suppressing appetite, improving blood sugar control, and promoting fat loss, GLP-1 helps create the conditions necessary for continued weight loss. When used under medical supervision and combined with a healthy diet, regular exercise, and behavior modification, GLP-1 therapy can provide the extra push needed to break through a plateau and achieve lasting weight loss success.

For those struggling with a weight loss plateau, incorporating GLP-1 therapy under medical supervision can provide the following benefits:

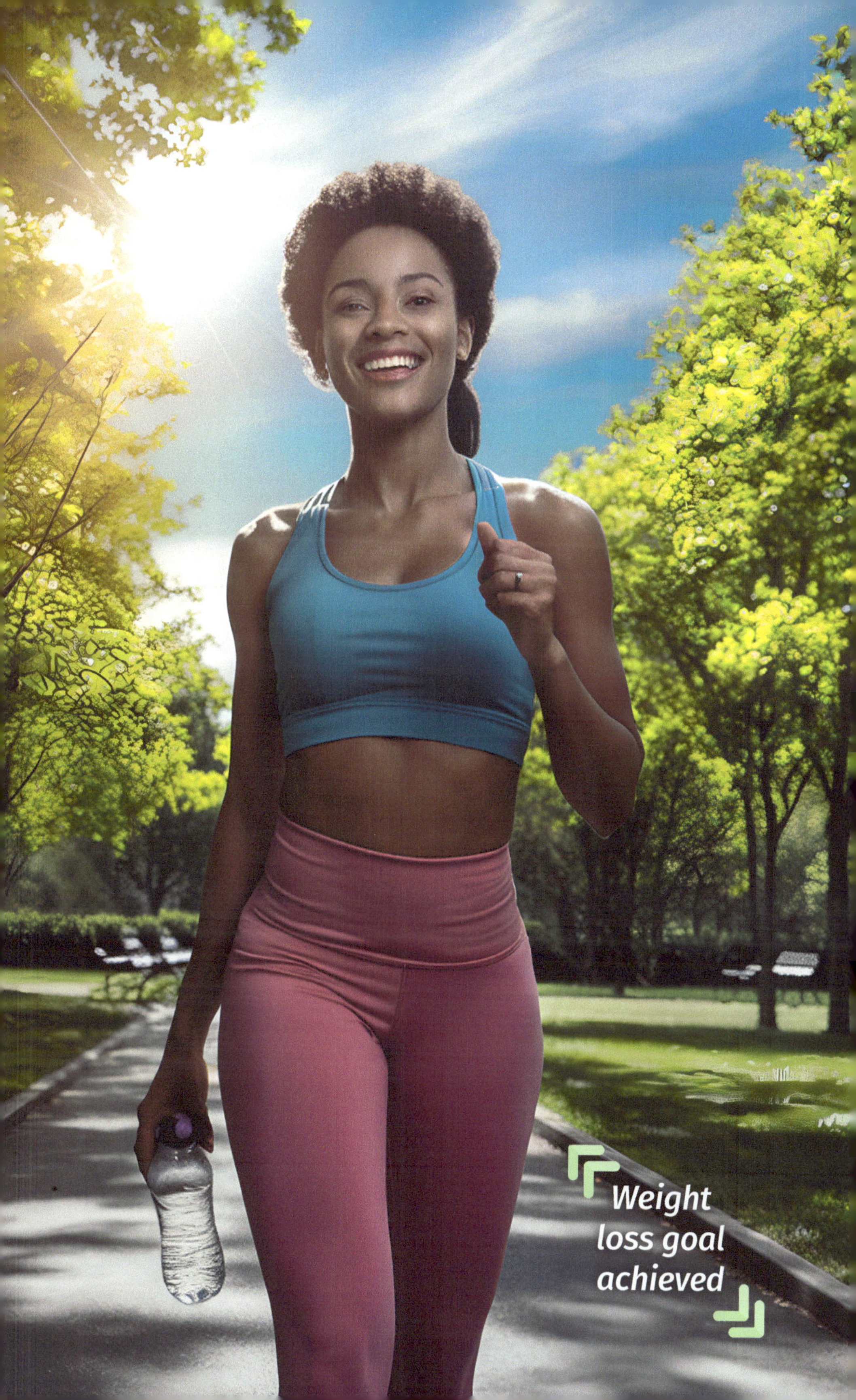
Weight
loss goal
achieved

> **Medical Consultation:** Discuss with one of our healthcare Providers to determine which GLP-1 therapy will be appropriate for you.

> **Medication Options:** Guidance will be provided on which GLP-1, dosage and administration that will be good for you.

> **Diet and Exercise Integration:** Continue following a balanced, reduced-calorie diet and regular exercise routine. GLP-1 therapy should complement these efforts, not replace them.

> **Monitoring and Adjustments:** Regular follow-ups are essential to monitor progress, adjust dosages if necessary, and address any side effects.

> **Behavioral Support:** One of our Providers will counsel you and provide support on dietary and behavioral changes. This can enhance the effectiveness of GLP-1 therapy.

In the face of challenges, persistence is your greatest ally. When you feel like giving up, remember why you started and push forward with renewed determination.

Other Factors that can affect your weight loss goals

There are several factors that can contribute to a person not losing weight, even when they are making efforts through diet and exercise. Understanding these factors and implementing targeted strategies can help overcome these obstacles. Here are common factors and suggestions to help:

Factors Contributing to your inability to lose weight:

Hormonal Imbalance

> When your hormones are not optimized, due to menopause or Andropause, it can be difficult to lose weight

> Discuss with one of our esteemed healthcare providers to have your hormones checked. Critical hormones to check are Estrogen, Progesterone, Testosterone, T3, T4, A1C, Thyroid antibodies and Cortisol.

Chronic Stress

> Chronic stress increases cortisol levels, which can lead to weight gain, especially around the abdominal area.

> Practice stress-reducing techniques such as meditation, deep breathing exercises, yoga, or mindfulness.

Medical Conditions

> Conditions like hypothyroidism, Polycystic Ovary Syndrome (PCOS), and insulin resistance can make weight loss more difficult.

> Consult with a healthcare provider to manage underlying medical conditions and consider any necessary treatments or medications.

Medications

> Certain medications, such as antidepressants, antipsychotics, and corticosteroids, can cause weight gain.

> Discuss with your doctor the potential side effects of your medications and explore alternative treatments if possible.

Nutrient Deficiencies

> Deficiencies in essential nutrients like vitamin D, iron, and magnesium can affect metabolism and energy levels.

> Eat a balanced diet rich in fruits, vegetables, lean proteins, and whole grains. Consider supplementation if recommended by a healthcare provider.

Dehydration

> Inadequate water intake can affect metabolism and increase hunger.

> Drink at least 8 cups (2 liters) of water daily. Increase intake if you are physically active or live in a hot climate.

Overreliance on Processed Foods

> Consuming a diet high in processed foods can lead to weight gain due to high levels of sugar, unhealthy fats, and empty calories.

> Focus on whole, unprocessed foods. Prepare meals at home using fresh ingredients.

Inconsistent Eating Patterns

> Irregular mealtimes or frequent snacking can disrupt metabolism and lead to weight gain.

> Stick to a regular eating schedule with balanced meals and snacks. Ensure you eat enough protein.

Lack of Support

> Social isolation or lack of support can make weight loss more challenging.

> Seek support from friends, family, or weight loss groups. Consider working with a dietitian or personal trainer.

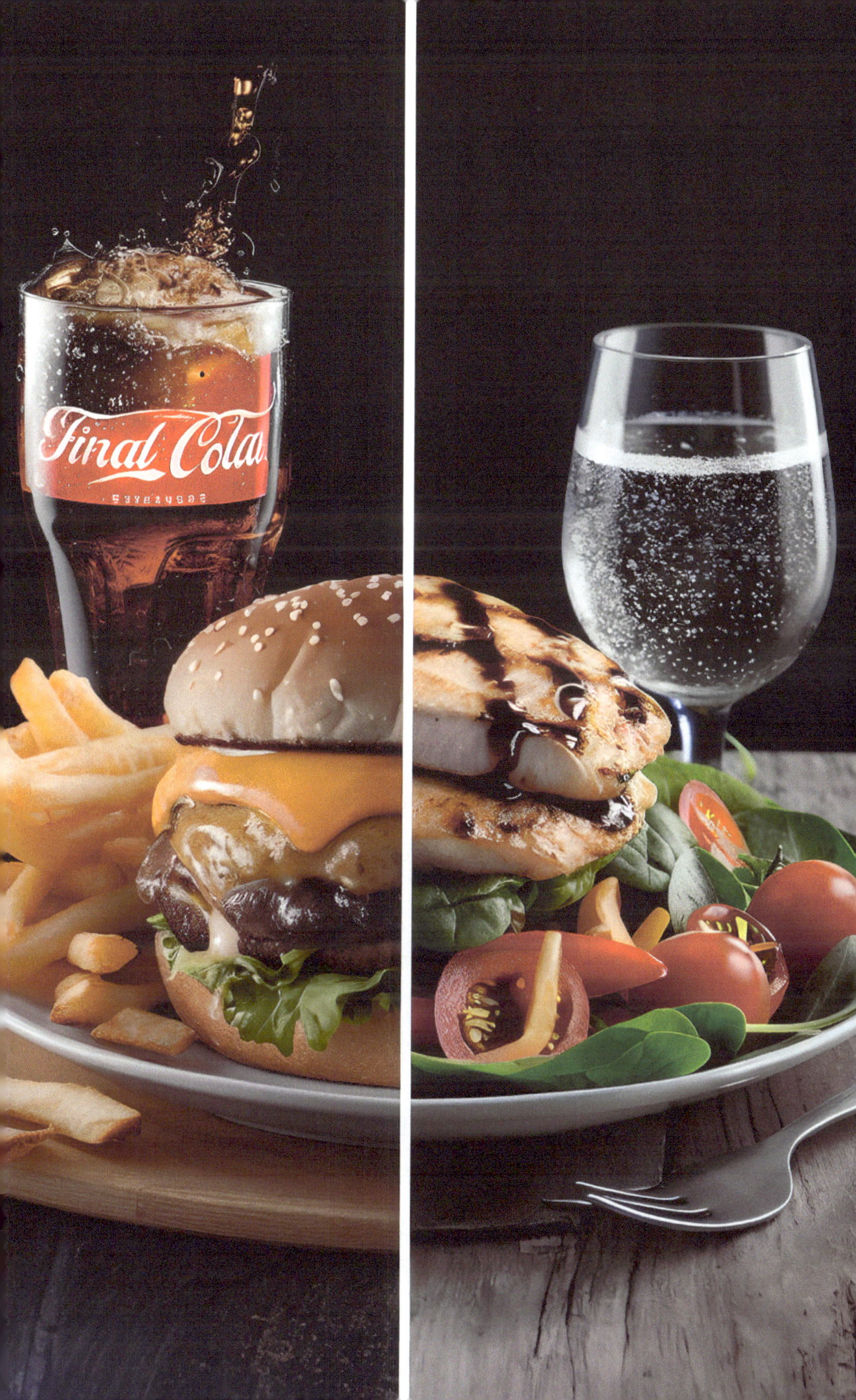
Final Cola

Maintenance Phase to lasting Weight loss

The Maintenance Phase of the Ultimate Guide to lasting Weight loss program is designed to help you sustain your weight loss and solidify the healthy habits you've developed throughout your journey.

This phase is crucial for ensuring that the weight you've lost stays off and that you continue to enjoy the benefits of a healthier lifestyle. During this phase, the focus shifts to maintaining your progress while gradually weaning off GLP-1 medications under professional guidance.

Weaning Off GLP-1

As you enter the Maintenance Phase, your healthcare provider will help you create a plan to gradually reduce and eventually discontinue the use of GLP-1 medications. This process is important to ensure your body adjusts smoothly without experiencing sudden changes in appetite or weight. Your provider will monitor your progress closely, adjusting your plan as needed to maintain stability and prevent weight regain.

Maintaining a New Lifestyle

The Maintenance Phase is all about incorporating the new, healthy habits you've learned into your daily life. Continue to focus on a balanced diet, rich in whole foods like fruits, vegetables, lean proteins, and whole grains. Keep your sodium and sugar intake low to support ongoing weight management and overall health. Regular exercise remains essential; aim for a mix of cardiovascular, strength training, and flexibility exercises to keep your body fit and strong.

Strategies to Maintain Lost Weight

1. Mindful Eating: Pay attention to hunger and fullness cues and avoid emotional or stress-related eating.

2. Portion Control: Keep portion sizes in check to avoid overeating.

3. Regular Meals: Stick to a routine of regular, balanced meals to prevent hunger-driven overeating.

4. Stay Active: Incorporate physical activity into your daily routine, aiming for at least 150 minutes of moderate exercise per week.

5. Hydration: Drink plenty of water throughout the day to stay hydrated and support metabolism.

6. Healthy Snacks: Choose nutritious snacks like nuts, fruits, and yogurt to keep energy levels stable between meals.

7. Monitor Progress: Regularly check your weight and body measurements to stay on track.

7. Support System: Engage with a support group or a health coach for motivation and accountability.

Continued Use of GLP-1

In the maintenance phase, you may require GLP-1 injections periodically, such as once every two weeks, once a month, or as needed, depending on how well you've maintained your weight. It's crucial not to wait until you've gained more than 10 pounds before taking action. If you notice weight gain, take steps to reduce it through diet and exercise, or seek help to restart GLP-1 injections as necessary. Keeping your weight down and well-maintained is important to avoid obesity and its associated complications.

For some individuals, continued use of GLP-1 medications might be recommended to help maintain weight loss. If your healthcare provider determines that ongoing use of GLP-1 is beneficial for you, it will be incorporated into your long-term maintenance plan. This approach can help manage appetite, improve satiety, and prevent weight regain. Regular follow-ups with your healthcare provider will ensure that the use of GLP-1 remains safe and effective for your individual needs.

Lifelong Commitment to Health

The Maintenance Phase is not just about keeping the weight off but embracing a lifelong commitment to your health. By continuing to make mindful food choices, staying active, and utilizing the support of your healthcare team, you can maintain your weight loss and enjoy a healthier, more vibrant life. Remember, the habits you've formed during the Ultimate Guide to lasting Weight loss program are the foundation for your ongoing success. Stay focused, stay motivated, and celebrate your achievements as you continue on your journey to wellness.

Success is the sum of small efforts repeated day in and day out. Keep going, keep growing, and you'll achieve more than you ever imagined.

Dining Out and On-the-Go Practical Tips

Maintaining a healthy diet while traveling, on the go, or on vacation can be particularly challenging. The temptation of fast food, the convenience of unhealthy snacks, and the allure of indulgent vacation meals can make it difficult to stick to nutritious choices.

Limited access to fresh foods, irregular meal schedules, and social pressures to indulge further complicate the task. However, with careful planning, mindful eating, and a commitment to making healthier choices, it is possible to navigate these challenges and maintain your dietary goals, even when you're away from home.

Dining out can be a challenge when trying to maintain a healthy diet, but with the right strategies and choices, it is possible to enjoy a meal out without derailing your dietary goals. Here are some guidelines for dining out, along with healthy options and foods to avoid:

Guidelines for Dining Out

Plan Ahead

> Research the restaurant menu online before you go.

> Helps you choose healthier options and avoid impulsive, less healthy choices.

Portion Control

> Restaurant portions are often larger than necessary.

> Prevents overeating.

> Tips: Consider sharing a dish, ordering a half-portion, or boxing up half of your meal to take home.

Start with a Salad

> Begin your meal with a garden salad with a light dressing.

> Reduces hunger and helps you eat less of the main course.

> Tips: Opt for dressings on the side and avoid high-calorie toppings like croutons and bacon.

Avoid Starters and Bread Baskets

> Skip high-calorie appetizers and bread baskets.

> Saves room for healthier, more balanced food choices.

Choose Grilled, Baked, or Steamed

> Opt for dishes that are grilled, baked, or steamed rather than fried or sautéed in heavy sauces.

> Reduces calorie and fat intake.

Focus on Protein and Vegetables

> Choose lean proteins like chicken, fish, or tofu, and pair them with plenty of vegetables.

> Ensures a balanced meal with essential nutrients.

Watch the Sauces and Dressings

> Request sauces and dressings on the side.

> Allows you to control the amount you consume, reducing added calories and unhealthy fats.

Limit Alcohol

> Alcohol can add empty calories and impair judgment about food choices.

> Helps maintain calorie control and overall health.

> Tips: If you choose to drink, opt for a glass of wine or a light beer, and limit yourself to one drink.

Stay Hydrated

> Drink plenty of water before and during your meal.

> Helps control hunger and aids digestion.

Mindful Eating

> Eat slowly and savor each bite.

> Helps you recognize when you're full and prevents overeating.

Healthy Options

Salads

> Mixed greens with grilled chicken, avocado, tomatoes, cucumbers, and a vinaigrette dressing on the side.

> Provides a variety of nutrients and is generally low in calories.

Grilled or Baked Fish

> Grilled salmon with steamed vegetables and quinoa.

> High in protein and omega-3 fatty acids.

Vegetable-Based Dishes

> Stir-fried vegetables with tofu or vegetable curry with brown rice.

> Rich in vitamins, minerals, and fiber.

Lean Proteins

> Grilled chicken breast with a side of steamed broccoli and a small baked sweet potato.

> Provides essential amino acids with low saturated fat.

Soups

> Broth-based soups like minestrone or vegetable soup.

> Low in calories and filling.

Whole Grains

> Quinoa salad with mixed vegetables and a light dressing.

> Provides fiber and complex carbohydrates.

Foods to Avoid

Fried Foods

> Fried chicken, French fries, onion rings.

> High in unhealthy fats and calories.

Creamy Sauces and Dressings

> Alfredo sauce, ranch dressing.

> High in calories and saturated fats.

High-Calorie Appetizers

> Mozzarella sticks, nachos, wings.

> Often high in fat and calories.

Sugary Beverages

> Sodas, sweetened iced teas, cocktails with sugary mixers.

> Provide empty calories and can lead to overeating.

Large Portions of Starches

> Large servings of pasta, rice, or potatoes.

> Can contribute to excess calorie intake.

Processed Meats

> Sausages, bacon, deli meats.

> High in sodium, unhealthy fats, and preservatives.

Desserts

> Cakes, pastries, ice cream.

> High in sugar and calories.

Healthy Dining Out Strategies

> Ask for Modifications: Don't be afraid to ask for modifications, such as steaming vegetables instead of sautéing them or serving sauces on the side.

> Opt for Clear Soups: Choose broth-based soups over creamy ones to save on calories.

> Skip the Sugar: Request no added sugar in beverages or dressings.

> Balance Your Plate: Aim to fill half your plate with vegetables, a quarter with lean protein, and a quarter with whole grains.

> Avoid All-You-Can-Eat Buffets: These can lead to overeating; opt for à la carte options instead.

By following these guidelines and making mindful choices, you can enjoy dining out while still staying on track with your health and weight loss goals.

Healthy Fast-Food and Snack Options

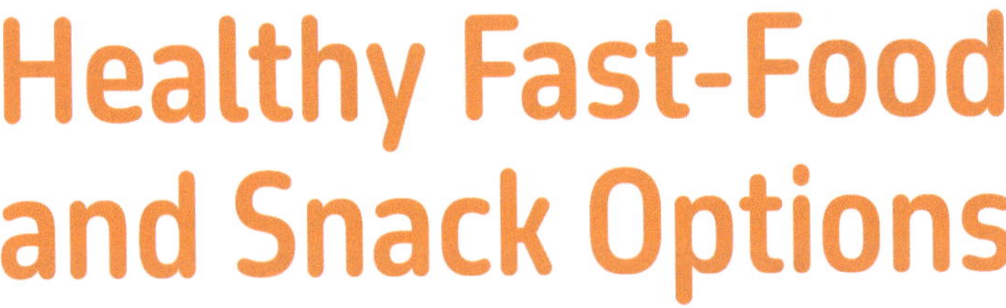

For anyone looking to maintain a healthy diet while on the road, it can be challenging to find nutritious options at fast food restaurants. However, with careful choices, it's possible to enjoy a meal or snack that is both satisfying and conducive to weight loss. Here are healthy fast-food and snack options with their approximate calorie counts:

1. Grilled Chicken Sandwich
- Restaurants: Chick-fil-A, Wendy's, McDonald's
- Calories: ~350-450 calories (without mayo or high-calorie sauces)

2. Salad with Grilled Protein
- Restaurants: Panera Bread, Chipotle, Wendy's
- Calories: ~300-500 calories (depending on toppings and dressing)

3. Burrito Bowl
- Restaurants: Chipotle, Qdoba, Taco Bell
- Calories: ~400-600 calories (without rice, tortilla, or sour cream)

4. Grilled Chicken Wrap
- Restaurants: Chick-fil-A, Wendy's, Subway
- Calories: ~350-450 calories (depending on sauces and toppings)

5. Egg White Breakfast Sandwich
- Restaurants: Starbucks, Dunkin', Subway
- Calories: ~250-350 calories

6. Fresh Fruit and Yogurt Parfait
- Restaurants: McDonald's, Starbucks
- Calories: ~150-200 calories

7. Veggie Sandwich or Wrap
> Restaurants: Subway, Panera Bread
> Calories: ~300-400 calories (depending on bread and toppings)

8. Turkey or Chicken Salad
> Restaurants: Arby's, Panera Bread
> Calories: ~350-450 calories (without high-calorie dressings)

9. Grilled Fish Tacos
> Restaurants: Baja Fresh, Rubio's, Taco Bell (Fresco menu)
> Calories: ~200-300 calories per taco

10. Soup and Salad Combo
> Restaurants: Panera Bread, Subway
> Calories: ~300-450 calories (depending on soup and salad choices)

11. Lettuce-Wrapped Burgers
> Restaurants: In-N-Out Burger, Five Guys
> Calories: ~300-450 calories (depending on toppings)

12. Grilled Chicken Nuggets
> Restaurants: Chick-fil-A
> Calories: ~130 calories (8-count)

13. Smoothies (Low-Sugar)
> Restaurants: Smoothie King, Jamba Juice
> Calories: ~200-300 calories (for small, low-sugar options)

14. Apple Slices or Fresh Fruit
> Restaurants: McDonald's, Chick-fil-A, Subway
> Calories: ~15-50 calories

15. Greek Yogurt with Nuts
> Restaurants: Starbucks, McDonald's
> Calories: ~200-250 calories

These calorie counts are approximate and can vary based on the specific restaurant and preparation. Be sure to check nutritional information from the restaurant directly whenever possible to make the best choices for your weight loss goals.

Tips for On-the-Go options:

> Plan Ahead: Know the menu options of common fast-food chains you'll encounter on your route and plan your meals accordingly.

> Avoid Sugary Drinks: Opt for water, unsweetened iced tea, or black coffee to save on calories.

> Portion Control: Fast food portions are often large. Consider ordering from the kid's menu or saving half of your meal for later.

> Mind the Sides: Swap out fries and chips for healthier sides like fruit, side salads, or yogurt.

> Stay Active: Even on the road, try to incorporate short walks or stretching exercises during breaks to stay active.

By choosing these healthier options, you can enjoy convenient meals without derailing you're your weight loss goals.

Conclusion
Your Path to Lifelong Health and Wellness

Congratulations on taking the first steps toward a healthier, happier you. "The Ultimate Guide to Lasting Weight Loss" is designed to be your steadfast companion on this transformative journey, providing you with the knowledge, tools, and support necessary to achieve and maintain your weight loss goals.

Throughout this guide, we've explored the four distinct phases of our program—Detox, Modified Ketogenic, Regular, and Maintenance. Each phase is meticulously crafted to ensure a smooth and effective transition from cleansing your body to adopting a sustainable, healthy lifestyle. By following the dietary guidelines, engaging in regular exercise, and incorporating behavior modification techniques, you have the foundation to build lasting healthy habits.

We've highlighted the powerful role of GLP-1 in overcoming weight loss plateaus, helping you achieve your goals more efficiently. Understanding how to utilize this hormone safely under the guidance of healthcare professionals can be a game-changer in your weight loss journey.

The Maintenance Phase is crucial for ensuring that the weight you lose stays off. This phase focuses on maintaining the new lifestyle habits you've developed, including balanced eating, regular physical activity, and ongoing behavior modification. Learning how to navigate dining out, manage occasional indulgences, and stay motivated is essential for long-term success.

We've provided you with practical tips for dining out, strategies for managing plateaus, and sample menus to keep your meals varied, satisfying, and aligned with your weight loss goals. These resources are designed to make your journey easier and more enjoyable, ensuring you have the support you need every step of the way.

Remember, this journey is not about perfection but about progress. Each healthy choice you make, each step you take, brings you closer to the vibrant, energetic life you deserve. Embrace the small victories

and learn from the challenges. Your persistence and dedication will lead to lasting change.

As you move forward, keep the vision of your healthiest self in mind. Use the tools and strategies provided in this guide to stay on track, even when faced with obstacles. Surround yourself with a supportive community, seek guidance from healthcare professionals when needed, and most importantly, believe in your ability to succeed.

"The Ultimate Guide to Lasting Weight Loss" is more than just a program—it's a commitment to yourself and your well-being. With determination, consistency, and the right support, you can achieve lasting weight loss and enjoy a lifetime of health and happiness.

Thank you for entrusting us with your journey. Here's to your success, your health, and a future filled with vitality. You've got this!

APPENDIX A

Quick Start Guide to A Slim and Healthy You In 4 Weeks!

WEEK 1

❯ Start the DETOX program

❯ Don't forget to drink a tablespoon of lemon juice and Apple Cider Vinegar mixed in at least 8oz of water

❯ Drink up to 80oz of water per day

❯ Eat very lean meats and plenty of fruits and veggies

❯ Take your weekly GLP-1 injection if qualified and approved by your healthcare provider

❯ Make sure you take your Detox Supplements as recommended

WEEK 2

❯ Start KETOSIS this week. (Eat Proteins Only)

❯ Eat Proteins Only for 4 days

❯ Drink up to one gallon of fluid per day

❯ Take your weekly Semaglutide or Tirzepatide injection

❯ Add your fruits and veggies this week on 5th day

❯ Start to get some daily activity

❯ Make sure you take your fat burner and multivitamin

WEEK 3

❯ We are on the way now

❯ Follow the previous instructions and you will continue to lose weight

❯ Do not eat if you are not hungry

❯ Drink up to one gallon of fluids per day

❯ Continue with your weekly injection.

❯ Report any signs of cravings, hunger or side effects

❯ Continue with daily physical activity

❯ Make sure you take your fat burner and multivitamin

WEEK 4

❯ Congratulations! If you follow the above program, you should have lost 10 to 20 pounds.

❯ Continue to follow our ultimate guide and a Slim and healthy body will be yours as a right and no more a privilege.

Every healthy choice you make is a victory in itself.

APPENDIX B

Two-Week Low Carb Sample Menu (1500 Calories per Day) Women are allowed between 1000 to 1200 calories and Men are allowed no more than 1500 calories.

WEEK 1

DAY 1

Breakfast:
• 2 scrambled eggs with spinach and feta cheese (200 calories)
• 1/2 avocado (120 calories)
• Black coffee or tea (0 calories)

Total: 320 calories

Snack:
• 1 small apple (80 calories)

Lunch:
• Grilled chicken salad with mixed greens, cherry tomatoes, cucumber, and olive oil vinaigrette (300 calories)
Total: 300 calories

Snack:
• 10 almonds (70 calories)

Dinner:
• Baked salmon with a side of steamed broccoli and cauliflower (350 calories)
Total: 350 calories

Snack:
• 1 cup Greek yogurt (unsweetened) with a handful of blueberries (150 calories)

DAILY TOTAL: 1270 CALORIES

DAY 2

Breakfast:
• Greek yogurt parfait with 1 cup Greek yogurt, 1/4 cup mixed berries, and 1 tablespoon chia seeds (220 calories)
Total: 220 calories

Snack:
• 1 small carrot with 2 tablespoons hummus (90 calories)

Lunch:
• Turkey lettuce wraps with avocado, tomato, and mustard (300 calories)
Total: 300 calories

Snack:
• 1 string cheese (80 calories)

Dinner:
• Beef stir-fry with bell peppers, broccoli, and soy sauce (350 calories)
Total: 350 calories

Snack:
• 1 ounce dark chocolate (120 calories)

DAILY TOTAL: 1160 CALORIES

DAY 3

Breakfast:
• Omelet with mushrooms, bell peppers, and cheddar cheese (250 calories)
Total: 250 calories

Snack:
• 1 small pear (80 calories)

Lunch:
• Spinach salad with grilled shrimp, avocado, and lemon vinaigrette (320 calories)
Total: 320 calories

Snack:
• 1/4 cup walnuts (150 calories)

Dinner:
• Zucchini noodles with marinara sauce and ground turkey (350 calories)
• Total: 350 calories

Snack:
• Cottage cheese with sliced strawberries (150 calories)

DAILY TOTAL: 1300 CALORIES

DAY 4

Breakfast:
• Chia pudding made with almond milk and topped with raspberries (200 calories)
Total: 200 calories

Snack:
• 1 boiled egg (70 calories)

Lunch:
• Chicken Caesar salad (300 calories)
Total: 300 calories

Snack:
• 1 small orange (60 calories)

Dinner:
• Pork tenderloin with roasted Brussels sprouts and carrots (350 calories)
Total: 350 calories

Snack:
• 1 small apple with 1 tablespoon almond butter (170 calories)

DAILY TOTAL: 1150 CALORIES

DAY 5

Breakfast:
• Smoothie with spinach, kale, avocado, and unsweetened almond milk (200 calories)
Total: 200 calories

Snack:
• 1 ounce almonds (160 calories)

Lunch:
• Tuna salad with mixed greens and olive oil (300 calories)
Total: 300 calories

Snack:
• 1 small cucumber with 2 tablespoons guacamole (80 calories)

Dinner:
• Baked cod with a side of asparagus and cherry tomatoes (350 calories)
Total: 350 calories

Snack:
• 1/2 cup berries with 1 tablespoon whipped cream (70 calories)

DAILY TOTAL: 1160 CALORIES

DAY 6

Breakfast:
• Scrambled eggs with bell peppers and onions (200 calories)
Total: 200 calories

Snack:
• 1 small plum (30 calories)

Lunch:
• Greek salad with feta cheese, olives, and grilled chicken (320 calories)
Total: 320 calories

Snack:
• 1/4 cup sunflower seeds (160 calories)

Dinner:
• Grilled steak with sautéed spinach and mushrooms (350 calories)
Total: 350 calories

Snack:
• 1 cup Greek yogurt (unsweetened) with a few slices of kiwi (150 calories)

DAILY TOTAL: 1210 CALORIES

DAY 7

Breakfast:
• Cottage cheese with sliced cucumber and tomato (200 calories)
Total: 200 calories

Snack:
• 1 boiled egg (70 calories)

Lunch:
• Salmon and avocado salad (300 calories)
Total: 300 calories

Snack:
• 1 small pear (80 calories)

Dinner:
• Chicken breast with roasted sweet potatoes and green beans (350 calories)
Total: 350 calories

Snack:
• 1 ounce dark chocolate (120 calories)

DAILY TOTAL: 1120 CALORIES

DAY 8

Breakfast:
• Greek yogurt with sliced almonds and a few raspberries (200 calories)
Total: 200 calories

Snack:
• 1 small apple (80 calories)

Lunch:
• Chicken and avocado lettuce wraps (320 calories)
Total: 320 calories

Snack:
• 1 ounce walnuts (150 calories)

Dinner:
• Shrimp stir-fry with broccoli and bell peppers (350 calories)
Total: 350 calories

Snack:
• 1/2 avocado (120 calories)

DAILY TOTAL: 1220 CALORIES

Healthy eating is a form of self-respect. Nourish your body, fuel your dreams, and watch yourself flourish.

DAY 9

Breakfast:
• Omelet with spinach, tomatoes, and goat cheese (250 calories)
Total: 250 calories

Snack:
• 1 small orange (60 calories)

Lunch:
• Turkey salad with mixed greens and balsamic vinaigrette (300 calories)
Total: 300 calories

Snack:
• 1/4 cup pistachios (160 calories)

Dinner:
• Grilled chicken with steamed zucchini and squash (350 calories)
Total: 350 calories

Snack:
• 1 cup Greek yogurt with blueberries (150 calories)

DAILY TOTAL: 1270 CALORIES

DAY 10

Breakfast:
• Smoothie with spinach, kale, avocado, and coconut milk (200 calories)
Total: 200 calories

Snack:
• 1 boiled egg (70 calories)

Lunch:
• Tuna salad with mixed greens and olive oil (300 calories)
Total: 300 calories

Snack:
• 1 small carrot with 2 tablespoons hummus (90 calories)

Dinner:
• Baked salmon with asparagus and cherry tomatoes (350 calories)
• Total: 350 calories

Snack:
• 1 ounce dark chocolate (120 calories)

DAILY TOTAL: 1130 CALORIES

DAY 11

Breakfast:
• Scrambled eggs with mushrooms and cheese (200 calories)
Total: 200 calories

Snack:
• 1 small apple (80 calories)

Lunch:
• Grilled chicken Caesar salad (300 calories)
Total: 300 calories

Snack:
• 1 string cheese (80 calories)

Dinner:
• Beef stir-fry with bell peppers and broccoli (350 calories)
Total: 350 calories

Snack:
• Cottage cheese with sliced strawberries (150 calories)

DAILY TOTAL: 1160 CALORIES

DAY 12

Breakfast:
• Chia pudding made with almond milk and topped with raspberries (200 calories)
Total: 200 calories

Snack:
• 1 small cucumber with 2 tablespoons guacamole (80 calories)

Lunch:
• Spinach salad with grilled shrimp and lemon vinaigrette (320 calories)
Total: 320 calories

Snack:
• 1 small orange (60 calories)

Dinner:
• Pork tenderloin with roasted Brussels sprouts and carrots (350 calories)
Total: 350 calories

Snack:
• 1 ounce dark chocolate (120 calories)

DAILY TOTAL: 1130 CALORIES

DAY 13

Breakfast:
• Greek yogurt parfait with 1 cup Greek yogurt, 1/4 cup mixed berries, and 1 tablespoon chia seeds (220 calories)
Total: 220 calories

Snack:
• 1 small pear (80 calories)

Lunch:
• Chicken lettuce wraps with avocado and salsa (300 calories)
Total: 300 calories

Snack:
• 1 ounce almonds (160 calories)

Dinner:
• Grilled cod with a side of sautéed spinach and mushrooms (350 calories)
Total: 350 calories

Snack:
• 1 cup Greek yogurt with a few slices of kiwi (150 calories)

DAILY TOTAL: 1160 CALORIES

DAY 14

Breakfast:
• Smoothie with kale, avocado, unsweetened almond milk, and a scoop of protein powder (250 calories)
Total: 250 caloriess

Snack:
• 1 small apple (80 calories)

Lunch:
• Greek salad with feta cheese, olives, and grilled chicken (300 calories)
Total: 300 calories

Snack:
• 1/4 cup walnuts (150 calories)

Dinner:
• Baked chicken breast with roasted Brussels sprouts and sweet potatoes (350 calories)
Total: 350 calories

Snack:
• 1 ounce dark chocolate (120 calories)

DAILY TOTAL: 1250 CALORIES

APPENDIX C

Two-Week Low Carb Spanish Cuisine Sample Menu (1500 Calories per Day) Women are allowed between 1000 to 1200 calories and Men are allowed no more than 1500 calories.

WEEK 1

DAY 1

Desayuno (Breakfast):
• *Tortilla de Espinacas* (Spinach omelet with 2 eggs and 1/2 cup spinach): 220 calories)
• 1/4 avocado: 60 calories
Total: 280 calories

Merienda (Snack):
• 1 small apple (80 calories)

Almuerzo (Lunch):
• *Ensalada de Pollo con Aguacate y Pimientos* (Chicken salad with avocado and bell peppers): 350 calories
Total: 350 calories

Merienda (Snack):
• 10 almonds (70 calories)

Cena (Dinner):
• *Bacalao al Horno* (Baked cod) with a side of grilled zucchini: 350 calories
Total: 350 calories

Merienda (Snack):
• 1 cup Greek yogurt (unsweetened) with a few strawberries: 150 calories

DAILY TOTAL: 1280 CALORIES

DAY 2

Desayuno:
• *Huevos Revueltos con Jamón y Queso* (Scrambled eggs with ham and cheese): 250 calories
Total: 250 calories

Merienda:
• 1 small cucumber with 2 tablespoons of guacamole: 80 calories

Almuerzo:
• *Ensalada de Atún con Espinacas y Aceite de Oliva* (Tuna salad with spinach and olive oil): 320 calories
Total: 320 calories

Merienda:
• 1 string cheese (80 calories)

Cena:
• *Pollo a la Parrilla con Brócoli y Espárragos* (Grilled chicken with broccoli and asparagus): 350 calories
Total: 350 calories

Merienda:
• 1 ounce dark chocolate: 120 calories

DAILY TOTAL: 1200 CALORIES

DAY 3

Desayuno:
• *Yogur Griego con Nueces y Frambuesas* (Greek yogurt with nuts and raspberries): 220 calories
Total: 220 calories

Merienda:
• 1 small pear (80 calories)

Almuerzo:
• *Ensalada de Gambas con Aguacate y Tomate* (Shrimp salad with avocado and tomato): 350 calories
Total: 350 calories

Merienda:
• 1/4 cup walnuts (150 calories)

Cena:
• *Pimientos Rellenos de Carne* (Stuffed peppers with ground beef): 350 calories
• **Total: 350 calories**

Merienda:
• 1/2 cup berries with 1 tablespoon whipped cream: 70 calories

DAILY TOTAL: 1230 CALORIES

DAY 4

Desayuno:
• Tortilla Española con Cebolla y Pimientos (Spanish omelet with onions and bell peppers): 250 calories
Total: 250 calories

Merienda:
• 1 small orange: 60 calories

Almuerzo:
• *Ensalada de Pollo al Estilo Español con Aceite de Oliva y Limón* (Spanish-style chicken salad with olive oil and lemon): 320 calories
Total: 320 calories

Merienda:
• 1 ounce almonds: 160 calories

Cena:
• *Merluza a la Plancha con Espárragos* (Grilled hake with asparagus): 350 calories
Total: 350 calories

Merienda:
• 1 cup Greek yogurt with a few blueberries: 150 calories

DAILY TOTAL: 1210 CALORIES

DAY 5

Desayuno:
• *Smoothie de Espinacas y Aguacate con Leche de Almendras Sin Azúcar* (Spinach and avocado smoothie with unsweetened almond milk): 200 calories
Total: 200 calories

Merienda:
• 1 small apple: 80 calories

Almuerzo:
• *Ensalada de Atún con Aguacate y Pepino* (Tuna salad with avocado and cucumber): 300 calories)
Total: 300 calories

Merienda:
• 1 small carrot with 2 tablespoons hummus: 90 calories

Cena:
• *Pollo al Horno con Col Rizada y Zanahorias* (Baked chicken with kale and carrots): 350 calories
Total: 350 calories

Merienda:
• 1 ounce dark chocolate: 120 calories

DAILY TOTAL: 1140 CALORIES

DAY 6

Desayuno:
• *Huevos Cocidos con Espinacas y Queso* (Boiled eggs with spinach and cheese): 200 calories
Total: 200 calories

Merienda:
• 1 small plum (30 calories)

Almuerzo:
• *Ensalada de Gambas con Espinacas y Aceite de Oliva* (Shrimp salad with spinach and olive oil): 320 calories
Total: 320 calories

Merienda:
• 1/4 cup sunflower seeds (160 calories)

Cena:
• *Filete de Ternera con Brócoli al Vapor* (Beef steak with steamed broccoli): 350 calories
Total: 350 calories

Merienda:
• 1/2 cup Greek yogurt with sliced kiwi: 150 calories

DAILY TOTAL: 1190 CALORIES

DAY 7

Desayuno:
• *Yogur Griego con Rodajas de Pepino y Tomates Cherry* (Greek yogurt with cucumber slices and cherry tomatoes): 200 calories)
Total: 200 calories

Merienda:
• 1 boiled egg (70 calories)

Almuerzo:
• *Ensalada de Pollo con Aguacate y Pimientos* (Chicken salad with avocado and bell peppers): 320 calories
Total: 320 calories

Merienda:
• 1 small apple with 1 tablespoon almond butter: 170 calories

Cena:
• *Merluza al Horno con Espárragos y Zanahorias* (Baked hake with asparagus and carrots): 350 calories
Total: 350 calories

Merienda:
• 1 ounce dark chocolate: 120 calories

DAILY TOTAL: 1130 CALORIES

DAY 8

Desayuno:
• *Smoothie de Kale, Aguacate, Leche de Almendras Sin Azúcar y Proteína en Polvo* (Kale, avocado, almond milk smoothie with protein powder): 250 calories
Total: 250 calories

Merienda:
• 1 small pear: 80 calories

Almuerzo:
• *Ensalada de Pollo con Aguacate y Tomate* (Chicken salad with avocado and tomato): 320 calories
Total: 320 calories

Merienda:
• 1 ounce walnuts (150 calories)

Cena:
• *Filete de Ternera a la Parrilla con Espinacas y Champiñones* (Grilled beef steak with spinach and mushrooms): 350 calories
Total: 350 calories

Merienda:
• 1 cup Greek yogurt with a few blueberries: 150 calories

DAILY TOTAL: 1320 CALORIES

DAY 9

Desayuno:
• *Tortilla de Espinacas con Queso* (Spinach omelet with cheese): 250 calories
Total: 250 calories

Merienda:
• 1 small apple: 80 calories

Almuerzo:
• *Ensalada de Atún con Espinacas y Aguacate* (Tuna salad with spinach and avocado): 300 calorie
Total: 300 calories

Merienda:
• 1 string cheese: 80 calories

Cena:
• *Pollo al Horno con Brócoli y Pimientos* (Baked chicken with broccoli and bell peppers): 350 calories)
Total: 350 calories

Merienda:
• 1 ounce dark chocolate: 120 calories

DAILY TOTAL: 1180 CALORIES

DAY 10

Desayuno:
• *Yogur Griego con Nueces y Frambuesas* (Greek yogurt with nuts and raspberries): 220 calories
Total: 220 calories

Merienda:
• 1 small carrot with 2 tablespoons hummus: 90 calories

Almuerzo:
• *Ensalada de Pollo con Aguacate y Tomate* (Chicken salad with avocado and tomato): 320 calories
Total: 320 calories

Merienda:
• 1/4 cup pistachios: 160 calories

Cena:
• *Filete de Ternera con Espárragos y Champiñones* (Beef steak with asparagus and mushrooms): 350 calories
Total: 350 calories

Merienda:
• 1 ounce dark chocolate: 120 calories

DAILY TOTAL: 1260 CALORIES

DAY 11

Desayuno:
• *Tortilla de Calabacín y Queso* (Zucchini and cheese omelet): 250 calories
Total: 250 calories

Merienda:
• 1 small pear: 80 calories

Almuerzo:
• *Ensalada de Atún con Espinacas y Aceite de Oliva* (Tuna salad with spinach and olive oil): 320 calories
Total: 320 calories

Merienda:
• 1 ounce almonds: 160 calories

Cena:
• *Pollo al Horno con Brócoli y Col Rizada* (Baked chicken with broccoli and kale): 350 calories
Total: 350 calories

Merienda:
• 1 cup Greek yogurt with a few blueberries: 150 calorie

DAILY TOTAL: 1330 CALORIES

DAY 12

Desayuno:
• *Smoothie de Aguacate y Espinacas* (Avocado and spinach smoothie with unsweetened almond milk): 200 calories
Total: 200 calories

Merienda:
• 1 small apple: 80 calories

Almuerzo:
• *Ensalada de Gambas con Aguacate y Pepino* (Shrimp salad with avocado and cucumber): 320 calories
Total: 320 calories

Merienda:
• 1/4 cup walnuts: 160 calories

Cena:
• *Bacalao a la Plancha con Espárragos* (Grilled cod with asparagus): 350 calories
Total: 350 calories

Merienda:
• 1 ounce dark chocolate: 120 calories

DAILY TOTAL: 1230 CALORIES

DAY 13

Desayuno:
• *Yogur Griego con Almendras y Frambuesas* (Greek yogurt with almonds and raspberries): 220 calories
Total: 220 calories

Merienda:
• 1 small cucumber with 2 tablespoons guacamole: 80 calories

Almuerzo:
• *Ensalada de Pollo con Pimientos y Aceite de Oliva* (Chicken salad with bell peppers and olive oil): 350 calories
Total: 350 calories

Merienda:
• 1 ounce pistachios: 160 calories

Cena:
• *Pollo a la Parrilla con Brócoli y Espárragos* (Grilled chicken with broccoli and asparagus): 350 calories
Total: 350 calories

Merienda:
• 1 cup Greek yogurt with a few strawberries: 150 calories

DAILY TOTAL: 1210 CALORIES

DAY 14

Desayuno:
• *Tortilla de Espinacas con Queso* (Spinach omelet with cheese): 250 calories
Total: 250 caloriess

Merienda:
• 1 small apple: 80 calories

Almuerzo:
• *Ensalada de Gambas con Aguacate y Tomate* (Shrimp salad with avocado and tomato): 320 calories
Total: 320 calories

Merienda:
• 1 ounce almonds: 160 calories

Cena:
• *Merluza al Horno con Espárragos y Zanahorias* (Baked hake with asparagus and carrots): 350 calories
Total: 350 calories

Merienda:
• 1 ounce dark chocolate: 120 calories

DAILY TOTAL: 1280 CALORIES

APPENDIX D

Two-Week Vegetarian Sample Menu (1500 Calories per Day). Women are allowed between 1000 to 1200 calories and Men are allowed no more than 1500 calories.

WEEK 1

DAY 1

Breakfast:
• Spinach and Banana Smoothie with unsweetened almond milk: 200 calories
Total: 200 calories

Snack:
• 1 small apple (80 calories)

Lunch:
• Chickpea Salad with avocado and tomato: 350 calories
Total: 300 calories

Snack:
• 1 ounce almonds: 160 calories

Dinner:
• Spanish Omelet with Spinach: 350 calories
Total: 350 calories

Snack:
• 1 cup Greek yogurt (unsweetened) with a handful of blueberries (150 calories)

DAILY TOTAL: 1360 CALORIES

DAY 2

Breakfast:
• Greek Yogurt with Nuts and Raspberries: 220 calories
Total: 220 calories

Snack:
• 1 small orange: 60 calories

Lunch:
• Quinoa Salad with spinach and chickpeas: 350 calorie
Total: 350 calories

Snack:
• 1 small carrot with 2 tablespoons hummus: 90 calories

Dinner:
• Stuffed Peppers with brown rice and vegetables: 350 calories
Total: 350 calories

Snack:
• 1 ounce dark chocolate (120 calories)

DAILY TOTAL: 1190 CALORIES

DAY 3

Breakfast:
• Kale and Mango Smoothie with unsweetened almond milk: 200 calories
Total: 200 calories

Snack:
• 1 small pear (80 calories)

Lunch:
• Lentil Salad with avocado and cucumber: 320 calories
Total: 320 calories

Snack:
• 1/4 cup walnuts (150 calories)

Dinner:
• Tofu Stew with vegetables: 350 calories
• **Total: 350 calories**

Snack:
• 1 cup Greek yogurt with a few strawberries: 150 calories

DAILY TOTAL: 1260 CALORIES

DAY 4

Breakfast:
• Whole Grain Toast with avocado and tomato: 250 calories
Total: 250 calories

Snack:
• 1 small apple: 80 calories

Lunch:
• Tempeh Salad with spinach and walnuts: 350 calories
Total: 300 calories

Snack:
• 1 small cucumber with 2 tablespoons guacamole: 80 calories

Dinner:
• Pumpkin and Carrot Soup: 350 calories)
Total: 350 calories

Snack:
• 1 ounce dark chocolate: 120 calories

DAILY TOTAL: 1230 CALORIES

DAY 5

Breakfast:
• Greek Yogurt with Almonds and Blackberries: 220 calories
Total: 220 calories

Snack:
• 1 small pear: 80 calories

Lunch:
• Chickpea Salad with tomato and cucumber: 320 calories
Total: 320 calories

Snack:
• 1 ounce pumpkin seeds: 150 calories

Dinner:
• Vegetable Curry with Tofu: 350 calories
Total: 350 calories

Snack:
• 1 cup Greek yogurt with a few blueberries: 150 calories

DAILY TOTAL: 1370 CALORIES

DAY 6

Breakfast:
• Spinach and Pineapple Smoothie with unsweetened almond milk: 200 calories
Total: 200 calories

Snack:
• 1 small orange: 60 calories

Lunch:
• Lentil Salad with avocado and tomato: 320 calories)
Total: 320 calories

Snack:
• 1 ounce almonds: 160 calories

Dinner:
• Mushroom and Asparagus Omelet: 350 calories
Total: 350 calories

Snack:
• 1 ounce dark chocolate: 120 calories

DAILY TOTAL: 1230 CALORIES

DAY 7

Breakfast:
• Greek Yogurt with Fruits and Nuts: 220 calories)
Total: 220 calories

Snack:
• 1 small apple: 80 calories

Lunch:
• Quinoa Salad with vegetables and chickpeas: 350 calories
Total: 350 calories

Snack:
• 1 small cucumber with 2 tablespoons hummus: 80 calories)

Dinner:
• Stuffed Peppers with vegetables: 350 calories
Total: 350 calories

Snack:
• 1 cup Greek yogurt with a few berries: 150 calories)

DAILY TOTAL: 1230 CALORIES

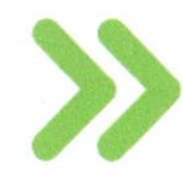

DAY 8

Breakfast:
• Kale and Mango Smoothie with unsweetened almond milk: 200 calories
Total: 200 calories

Snack:
• 1 small pear (80 calories)

Lunch:
• Chickpea Salad with spinach and avocado: 350 calories
Total: 350 calories

Snack:
• 1 ounce walnuts (150 calories)

Dinner:
• Tofu Stew with zucchini and tomato: 350 calories
Total: 350 calories

Snack:
• 1 cup Greek yogurt with a few blueberries: 150 calories

DAILY TOTAL: 1360 CALORIES

DAY 9

Breakfast:
• Greek Yogurt with Almonds and Raspberries: 220 calories
Total: 220 calories

Snack:
• 1 small apple: 80 calories

Lunch:
• Quinoa Salad with vegetables and chickpeas: 350 calories
Total: 350 calories

Snack:
• 1 ounce almonds: 160 calories

Dinner:
• Spinach and Mushroom Omelet: 350 calories
Total: 350 calories

Snack:
• 1 ounce dark chocolate: 120 calories

DAILY TOTAL: 1280 CALORIES

DAY 10

Breakfast:
• Spinach and Banana Smoothie with unsweetened almond milk: 200 calories
Total: 200 calories

Snack:
• 1 small orange: 60 calories

Lunch:
• Chickpea Salad with cucumber and tomato: 320 calories
Total: 320 calories

Snack:
• 1 ounce pumpkin seeds: 150 calories

Dinner:
• Stuffed Peppers with quinoa and vegetables: 350 calories
• **Total: 350 calories**

Snack:
• 1 cup Greek yogurt with a few berries: 150 calories

DAILY TOTAL: 1350 CALORIES

DAY 11

Breakfast:
• Greek Yogurt with Nuts and Blackberries: 220 calories
Total: 220 calories

Snack:
• 1 small pear: 80 calories

Lunch:
• Lentil Salad with avocado and cucumber: 320 calories
Total: 320 calories

Snack:
• 1 ounce almonds: 160 calories

Dinner:
• Tofu Stir-Fry with mixed vegetables: 350 calories
Total: 350 calories

Snack:
• 1 ounce dark chocolate: 120 calories

DAILY TOTAL: 1250 CALORIES

DAY 12

Breakfast:
• Kale and Mango Smoothie with unsweetened almond milk: 200 calories
Total: 200 calories

Snack:
• 1 small apple: 80 calories

Lunch:
• Chickpea Salad with spinach and avocado: 350 calories
Total: 350 calories

Snack:
• 1 ounce pumpkin seeds: 150 calories

Dinner:
• Vegetable Curry with tofu: 350 calories
Total: 350 calories

Snack:
• 1 cup Greek yogurt With a few strawberries: 150 calorie

DAILY TOTAL: 1380 CALORIES

DAY 13

Breakfast:
• Greek Yogurt with Almonds and Raspberries: 220 calories
Total: 220 calories

Snack:
• 1 small apple: 80 calories

Lunch:
• Lentil Salad with avocado and cucumber: 320 calories
Total: 320 calories

Snack:
• 1 ounce walnuts: 160 calories

Dinner:
• Stuffed Zucchini with quinoa and vegetables: 350 calories
Total: 350 calories

Snack:
• 1 cup Greek yogurt with a few blueberries: 150 calories

DAILY TOTAL: 1280 CALORIES

DAY 14

Breakfast:
• Spinach and Pineapple Smoothie with unsweetened almond milk: 200 calories
Total: 200 caloriess

Snack:
• 1 small pear: 80 calories

Lunch:
• Chickpea Salad with spinach and tomato: 350 calories
Total: 350 calories

Snack:
• 1 ounce almonds: 160 calories

Dinner:
• Vegetable Stir-Fry with tofu: 350 calories
Total: 350 calories

Snack:
• 1 ounce dark chocolate (120 calories)

DAILY TOTAL: 1310 CALORIES

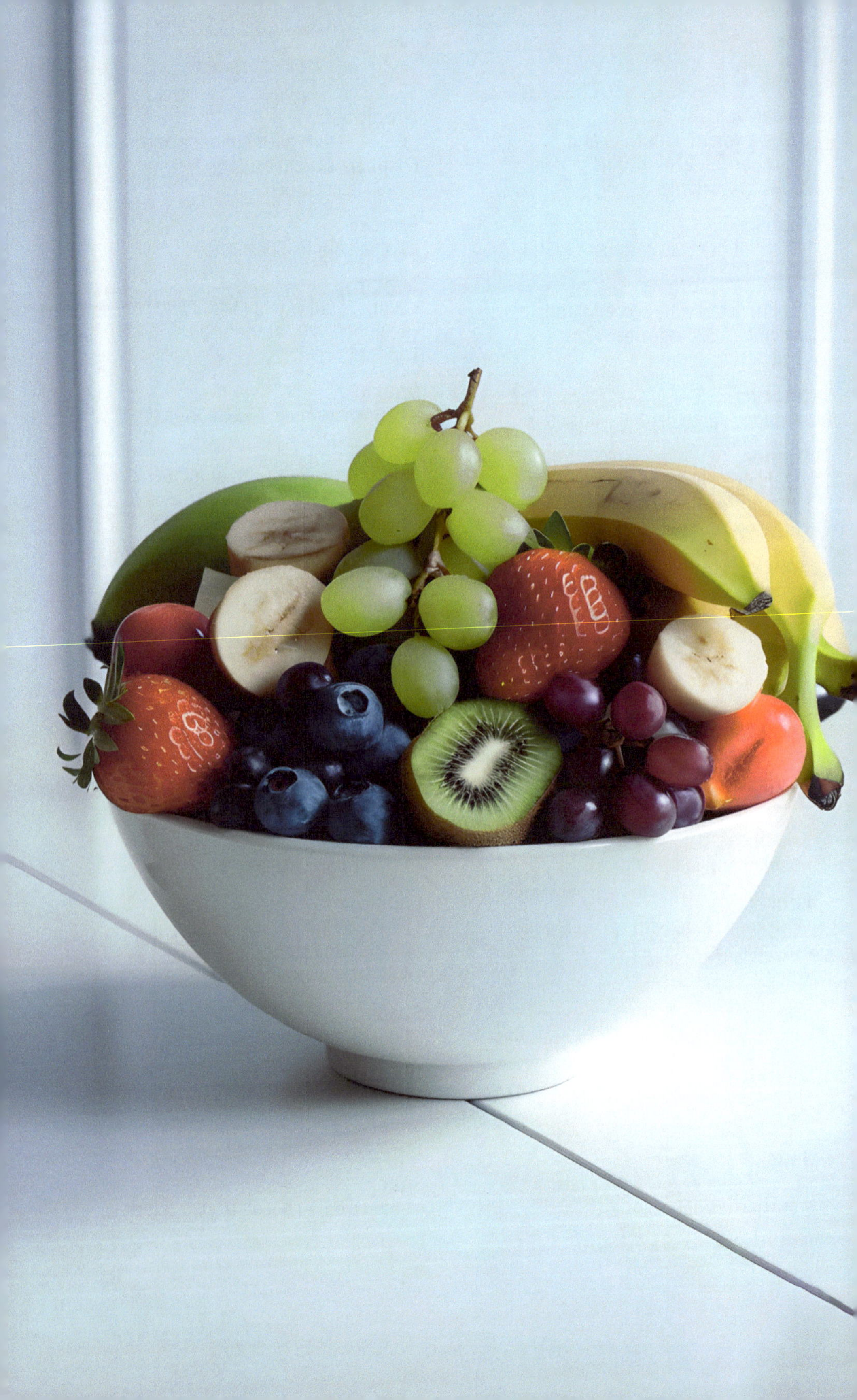

APPENDIX E
Healthy Salad Dressing Options

Choosing healthy salad dressings can significantly enhance the nutritional value of your salads without adding excessive calories, unhealthy fats, or sugars. Here are some healthy salad dressing options:

1. Olive Oil and Vinegar

> Ingredients: Extra virgin olive oil, balsamic vinegar, salt, and pepper.

> Benefits: Olive oil provides healthy monounsaturated fats and antioxidants, while vinegar can help with blood sugar regulation.

2. Lemon Vinaigrette

> Ingredients: Fresh lemon juice, extra virgin olive oil, Dijon mustard, minced garlic, salt, and pepper.

> Benefits: Low in calories and rich in vitamin C, this dressing is refreshing and light.

3. Greek Yogurt Dressing

> Ingredients: Greek yogurt, lemon juice, minced garlic, dill, salt, and pepper.

> Benefits: Greek yogurt adds creaminess without the fat, providing protein and probiotics.

4. Tahini Dressing

> Ingredients: Tahini (sesame seed paste), lemon juice, minced garlic, water, salt, and pepper.

> Benefits: Tahini is rich in healthy fats, vitamins, and minerals, and provides a nutty flavor.

5. Avocado Lime Dressing

> Ingredients: Ripe avocado, lime juice, cilantro, Greek yogurt, water, salt, and pepper.

> Benefits: Avocado provides healthy fats and fiber, while lime juice adds a zesty flavor.

6. Apple Cider Vinegar Dressing

❯ Ingredients: Apple cider vinegar, Dijon mustard, honey or maple syrup, extra virgin olive oil, salt, and pepper.

❯ Benefits: Apple cider vinegar can aid digestion, suppress appetite and has antibacterial properties.

7. Honey Mustard Dressing

❯ Ingredients: Dijon mustard, honey, apple cider vinegar, extra virgin olive oil, salt, and pepper.

❯ Benefits: This dressing is sweet and tangy, with a balance of healthy fats and natural sweetness.

8. Miso Dressing

❯ Ingredients: White miso paste, rice vinegar, sesame oil, honey, water, minced ginger, and garlic.

❯ Benefits: Miso provides probiotics, while sesame oil offers healthy fats and a rich flavor.

9. Cilantro Lime Dressing

❯ Ingredients: Fresh cilantro, lime juice, Greek yogurt, garlic, olive oil, salt, and pepper.

❯ Benefits: This dressing is packed with fresh herbs and vitamin C, adding a bright flavor to salads.

10. Pesto Dressing

❯ Ingredients: Fresh basil, pine nuts, Parmesan cheese, garlic, extra virgin olive oil, salt, and pepper.

❯ Benefits: Pesto is rich in healthy fats, vitamins, and minerals, adding a burst of flavor to any salad.

11. Raspberry Vinaigrette

❯ Ingredients: Fresh raspberries, balsamic vinegar, extra virgin olive oil, honey, salt, and pepper.

❯ Benefits: Raspberries provide antioxidants and a sweet-tart flavor.

12. Balsamic Vinaigrette

❯ Ingredients: Balsamic vinegar, extra virgin olive oil, Dijon mustard, honey, salt, and pepper.

❯ Benefits: A classic choice that is versatile and rich in antioxidants.

13. Sesame Ginger Dressing

❯ Ingredients: Sesame oil, rice vinegar, soy sauce or tamari, honey, minced ginger, and garlic.

❯ Benefits: This dressing offers a savory, Asian-inspired flavor with healthy fats and anti-inflammatory ginger.

14. Garlic Herb Dressing

❯ Ingredients: Extra virgin olive oil, lemon juice, minced garlic, chopped fresh herbs (like parsley, thyme, and rosemary), salt, and pepper.

❯ Benefits: Fresh herbs provide antioxidants and a burst of flavor.

15. Berry Balsamic Dressing

❯ Ingredients: Mixed berries (such as strawberries and blueberries), balsamic vinegar, olive oil, honey, salt, and pepper.

❯ Benefits: Combines the antioxidants from berries with the healthy fats from olive oil.

Tips for Healthy Salad Dressings

❯ Watch Portions: Even healthy dressings can add up in calories if used excessively. Stick to about 1-2 tablespoons per serving.

❯ Use Fresh Ingredients: Fresh herbs, citrus juices, and high-quality oils can make a big difference in flavor and nutrition.

❯ Avoid Added Sugars: Many store-bought dressings contain added sugars. Make your own to control the ingredients.

❯ Experiment with Flavors: Try different combinations of herbs, spices, and citrus to keep your salads interesting.

By choosing or making healthy salad dressings, you can enhance the flavor and nutritional profile of your salads, making them a more enjoyable and beneficial part of your diet.

About the Authors

Dr. Hilda Obi is a distinguished Doctor of Nursing Practice with a specialization in Obesity Medicine and a Certified Lifestyle and Wellness Consultant. She is also a Certified Women's Health Specialist, bringing a unique and comprehensive perspective to her practice. With over two decades of experience in the health and wellness industry, Dr. Hilda has dedicated her career to helping individuals achieve lasting weight loss and improve their overall health.

Dr. Hilda's approach is grounded in evidence-based practices and a holistic understanding of the human body. Her extensive background includes working with thousands of patients, guiding them through their weight loss journeys with compassion, expertise, and unwavering support. She is deeply committed to her patients' success, employing a blend of personalized nutrition plans, innovative medical treatments like GLP-1, and practical behavior modification strategies.

Dr. Hilda's dedication to her patients is deeply personal. She has faced her own health challenges, including a battle with thyroid cancer and her struggles with weight. These experiences have made her empathetic to the journeys of those she helps, understanding firsthand the physical and emotional hurdles that come with weight loss.

Dr. Hilda is happily married to her beloved husband, Victor Obi, and they have two amazing sons, both of whom are pursuing careers in the medical field. Her family's support and her personal health experiences drive her passion to help others achieve their own health and wellness goals.

In "The Ultimate Guide to Lasting Weight Loss," Dr. Hilda combines her medical expertise and years of hands-on experience to create a comprehensive guide that empowers readers to achieve their weight loss goals and maintain a healthy lifestyle. Her dedication to improving the lives of others is evident on every page of this transformative guide.

About the Co-Author

Victor Obi, co-author of "The Ultimate Guide to Lasting Weight Loss," is a highly experienced pharmacist with several years of expertise in the pharmaceutical health and wellness industry. His extensive knowledge in pharmacology and therapeutics plays a crucial role in understanding proper dosing, managing drug interactions, and ensuring the correct use of medications.

Victor's professional journey is marked by his dedication to improving patient outcomes through a comprehensive understanding of pharmaceutical treatments. His experience allows him to provide valuable insights into the safe and effective use of medications, an essential component for individuals on a weight loss journey, particularly those using medical treatments like GLP-1.

Victor's empathy and charitable nature extend beyond his professional life. He is deeply committed to helping others achieve their health and wellness goals, offering support and guidance with compassion and understanding. His ability to relate to patients' struggles and provide tailored solutions makes him an invaluable resource in the weight loss process.

In this book, Victor's contributions are instrumental in merging the medical and pharmaceutical perspectives, offering readers a well-rounded approach to weight loss. His expertise ensures that the guide is not only comprehensive but also safe and practical for everyday use.

Victor is happily married to Dr. Hilda Obi, and together they have two amazing sons pursuing careers in the medical field. His family's support and his commitment to patient care drive his passion for making a positive impact on the lives of those seeking a healthier lifestyle.

www.ingramcontent.com/pod-product-compliance
Lightning Source LLC
Chambersburg PA
CBHW042119150726
48005CB00026B/35